"While social media and technology have the potential to connect people in new ways, they also have the potential to deprive us of meaningful relationships and real connection. Tom Kersting is the go-to guy not only for explaining how technology is harmful to many of today's youth but also for providing a blueprint to help them escape the clutches of a social media culture that can rob them of what's truly important. I highly recommend this book to every parent, teacher, and leader."

Joel Comm, *New York Times* bestselling author

"Thomas Kersting sheds a powerful light on the negative impact digital overuse can have on children. Information is power, and this book is packed with alarming insight and practical advice for families who want a healthier balance and relationship with technology."

Rachel Campos-Duffy, FOX News contributor and host of *Moms* on FOXNation

"Nothing has changed the day-to-day life of modern American children more than smartphones and tablets. In *Disconnected*, Tom Kersting provides parents with an urgent wake-up call to the effects too much screen time can have on our children's social, emotional, and intellectual development. Tom's clinical research and experience, combined with his compassionate and practical solutions for families, makes *Disconnected* an insightful and necessary resource for moms and dads searching for answers. I have four boys under the age of fourteen, and if you're like me, trying to help each of your children have the proper balance between digital and real world experiences, *Disconnected* may be the most important book on parenting you'll read this year."

David Savage, cofounder of Content Watch Holdings, makers of Net Nanny® Parental Control Software

"*Disconnected* is more than a fact-checked indictment of the technology industry; it's a recovery manual for those most affected by the dark side of technology and a necessary guidebook of strategies for every parent, educator, and professional."

John Jolliffe, marriage and family therapist,
coexecutive producer of *Mack & Moxy*,
and former nationally syndicated radio personality

"*Disconnected* is a must-read for every parent. It is like taking a cold shower, waking you up to the reality of the digital epidemic threatening our children. Thomas Kersting sounds the alarm, warning how overindulgence of screen time plagues the emotional and psychological development of our children and society as a whole."

Tim Smith, founder/principal of The Smith Group

DISCONNECTED

How to Protect Your Kids from the Harmful
Effects of Device Dependency

THOMAS KERSTING

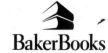

BakerBooks

a division of Baker Publishing Group
Grand Rapids, Michigan

Published by Baker Books
a division of Baker Publishing Group
PO Box 6287, Grand Rapids, MI 49516-6287
www.bakerbooks.com

Printed in the United States of America

Library of Congress Cataloging-in-Publication Data
Names: Kersting, Tom, 1972– author.
Title: Disconnected : how to protect your kids from the harmful effects of device
    dependency / Thomas Kersting.
Description: Grand Rapids, Michigan : Baker Books, a division of Baker Publishing
    Group, [2020]
Identifiers: LCCN 2020003243 | ISBN 9781540900302 (paperback)
Subjects: LCSH: Internet addiction in adolescence. | Internet—Physiological effect. |
    Internet—Psychological aspects. | Internet and teenagers. | Parenting.
Classification: LCC RJ506.I58 K47 2020 | DDC 616.85/8400835—dc23
LC record available at https://lccn.loc.gov/2020003243

The author is represented by the literary agency of Park & Fine Literary and Media.

Some names and details have been changed to protect the privacy of the individuals involved.

20 21 22 23 24 25 26   7 6 5 4 3 2 1

I would like to thank my beautiful wife
and two wonderful children for all their support
and encouragement in everything I do.

CONTENTS

INTRODUCTION

I was a helmetless, Big Wheel–riding child of the 1980s. I walked a half mile in the dark to the bus stop each morning, faced the occasional bully, threw eggs at other kids on Halloween, and rode my Huffy all around town when I was ten. I played tackle football with no pads and baseball without a heart protector. I sat in the back seat of my mom's Ford Granada without wearing a seat belt. I was outside all day long in the summer along with the other kids in my neighborhood. Nothing was planned out for us, and the only thing we cared about was adventure. We had Ataris and Nintendos but spent much less time playing them than we did playing outside with each other. Handheld devices did not exist, so my friends and I were never distracted from the fun we had together. When it was time for dinner, we were home on time and ate with our families—every night. We had few worries and were just, well, kids. And we all survived.

Today, my greatest source of pride is fatherhood. It is the most rewarding thing in the world but also the most frightening. The world I once lived in as a child is much different from the one my children live in today. In many ways this is a good thing. My kids always wear their seatbelts, never get on their bikes without a helmet, and do not throw eggs at other kids on Halloween. Yet the dangers you and I faced as children pale in comparison to the one our kids are facing. This danger is changing the very meaning of what it means to be a kid and even what it means to be a human—and this danger is wounding our children's mental, emotional, and social health like nothing we've seen before.

Several years ago my family and I enjoyed a wonderful trip out West. We visited a number of national parks including Yellowstone, Bryce Canyon, and Zion. It was the vacation of a lifetime. The flight back home to LaGuardia Airport in New York was long, and I remember feeling eager to exit the plane, get through baggage claim, and arrive home. When we finally disembarked and started making our way through the terminal, I stopped in my tracks. I felt like I had just entered the Twilight Zone. Screens were everywhere, and not just in the palms of the people I passed. Flashing tablets loaded with social media apps and games were perfectly positioned in front of every barstool and restaurant seat. I've spent a fair amount of my life in airports, and I'd met people from all around the world and learned so much while sipping a beer from one of those stools. The airport had replaced these experiences with machines. At the time of our trip, I had been speaking for several years to parent groups about the negative effect that too much technology was having on our children's well-being, so I was ahead of the curve, but this experience was different—this was technology on steroids.

As our family continued our long walk to the baggage claim area, I felt helpless. I hoped that what I witnessed was an isolated case, limited to the terminal we had flown into, but it wasn't. As we walked past more restaurants, bars, and waiting areas, the scene was the same—nearly everyone was connected to a screen and disconnected from each other. Strangers remained strangers.

Although I was reaching a lot of people through lectures, counseling sessions, and television appearances, I knew I had to do more to help parents understand the challenges their children will face in our hyperconnected world. That is why I wrote this book. It is a call to action.

The cold hard fact is this: *our children do not have control over electronic devices and screens; electronic devices and screens have control over them.* Much of what you will read in the coming pages is fascinating and also frightening, but if you stick with me you will see the light at the end of the tunnel. I'll share with you real-life stories from my experiences as a private practice therapist and public school counselor. I've also included scientific evidence and research-based studies to support my claims, along with valuable tips at the end of each chapter.

Screens are the cause of many of our children's problems, ranging from anxiety disorders to family problems to school and social problems. Unplugging our children and ourselves will not be easy, but it is possible. And in the final section of the book I provide a host of strategies you can utilize to help pull your family away from the screens and closer to each other.

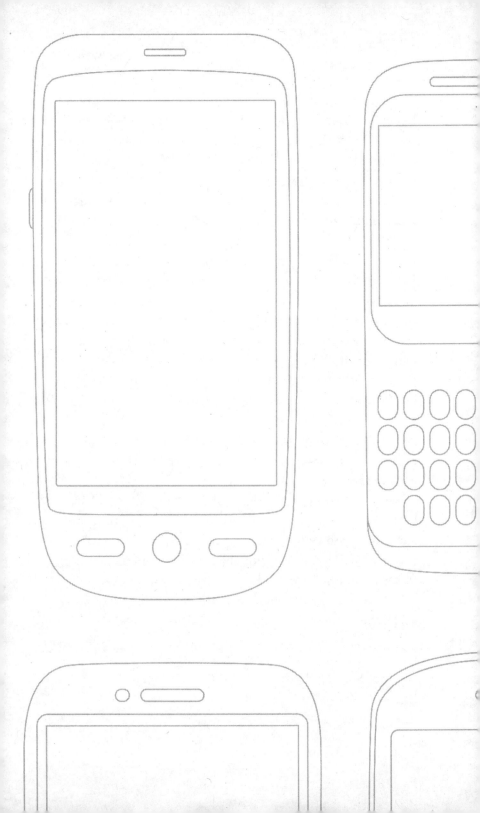

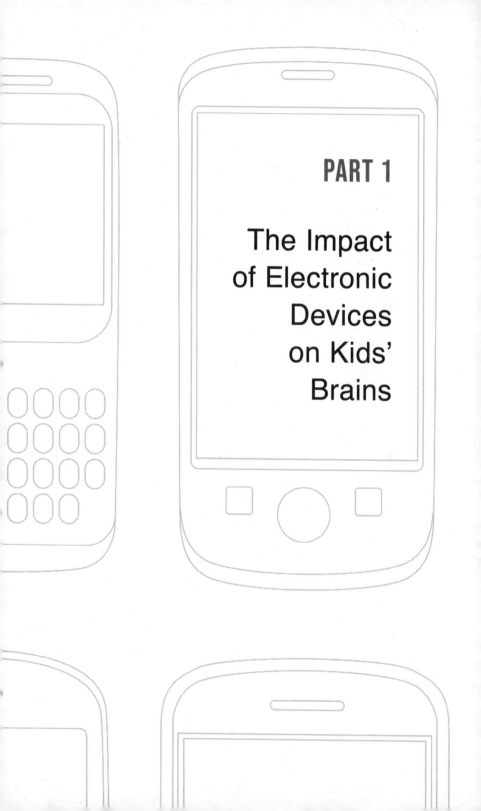

PART 1

The Impact of Electronic Devices on Kids' Brains

CHAPTER 1

Our Changing Reality

Acquired ADHD, Anxiety, and Neuroplasticity

Since 2002 I've been a member of the Intervention & Referral Services (I&RS) committee at a local high school where I work as a counselor. The role of the committee is to provide academic accommodations to students with temporary or permanent disabilities when there is evidence that the disability is affecting the student's learning. Some common disabilities the committee has reviewed over the years include concussions, diabetes, Crohn's disease, and specific learning issues.

During the 2009 school year, I noticed the types of disabilities referred to I&RS had started to change. We began receiving countless referrals for teenage students diagnosed with Attention Deficit Hyperactivity Disorder (ADHD). ADHD is a neurological condition that causes a combination of the following symptoms: inattention, disorganization and lack of focus, and sometimes impulsivity and hyperactivity. These symptoms are very noticeable by age five, and the average age at diagnosis is eight years old. Strangely, these referrals were for fourteen- and fifteen-year-olds newly diagnosed with the disorder.

As a school counselor by day and private practice therapist by night, I had twenty-plus years of experience working with ADHD children and their families. This sudden influx of attention deficit teenagers didn't make sense to me. Was it possible that this many parents and teachers had missed all the symptoms when these kids were in elementary or middle school? How could this many kids possibly have slipped through the cracks?

I started to aggressively research this new ADHD phenomenon and even consulted with neighboring school districts. My colleagues were also seeing precisely what I was—an exorbitant number of teenagers being diagnosed with the disorder. My research led me to the work of Dr. Gary Small, professor of psychiatry and director of the UCLA Longevity Center at the Semel Institute for Neuroscience and Human Behavior. Dr. Small is one of the world's top innovators in science and technology. In 2007 Small began researching technology's impact on the brain and discovered that when research subjects spent as little as an hour a day online, the activity patterns in their brains changed dramatically. According to Small, "The human brain is malleable, always changing in response to its environment."[1] He explains how sensitive the brain actually is. The many pieces of information the brain takes in, in the form of sights, sounds, feelings, and other experiences, causes a complex cascade of neurochemical electrical consequences. With repeated stimuli the neural circuits in the brain become excited, and if other neural circuits are neglected they will be weakened. A young person's brain, which is still developing, is particularly sensitive to the stimulations offered by modern technology.

Dr. Small discovered that kids' time on powerful electronic devices was actually changing their brains, something known as *neuroplasticity*. Neuroplasticity is the brain's ability to reorganize itself by forming new neural connections, leaving behind past traits and developing new ones. Could all of this screen time, in changing kids' brains, cause older children to display inattentiveness, lack of focus, and disorganization— all symptoms of ADHD? Yes. According to Dr. Elias Aboujaoude, director of Stanford University's Impulse Control Disorders Clinic, "The more we become used to just sound bites and tweets, the less patient we will become with more complex, more meaningful information. And I do think we might lose the ability to analyze things with any depth and nuance. Like any skill, if you don't use it you lose it."[2]

Dr. John Ratey, Clinical Professor of Psychiatry at Harvard Medical School, has coined the term *acquired attention deficit disorder*, describing how screen time was rewiring kids' brains.[3] The word *acquired* fascinated me because it meant that potentially thousands of teenagers were being misdiagnosed with a disorder they might not have and were often being prescribed powerful medication for. I decided to dig a little deeper with my caseload of recently diagnosed ADHD students at the high school. I gathered records and notes from their elementary and middle school counselors and teachers and, as I had suspected, I couldn't find any evidence of ADHD symptoms at earlier stages in their education.

Although Dr. Small's research is too new to be conclusive, he believes that in addition to attention deficit symptoms, too much time online might cause a host of other issues ranging from trouble maintaining eye contact to difficulty interacting with others. And in the decade since Dr. Small's groundbreaking research, many other studies have come out that link excessive screen time to anxiety, depression, and behavioral issues. One such study, conducted by Dr. Michael Van Ameringen, evaluated 254 freshmen at McMaster University in Ontario, Canada. Thirty-three of the students met criteria for internet addiction while 107 met the criteria for problematic internet use. The students' mental health was also assessed during the study, and those who met the criteria for internet addiction showed higher rates of inattention, impulsivity, anxiety, and depression.[4]

The implications of this research have lined up with my experiences working with teens as I have seen an incredible increase in attention problems and mental health issues. Recently I spoke to the freshman health classes at my high school about mental health. There were a total of nine classes, and the teachers were doing a lesson on teen depression and suicide. The lesson started with a short video followed by a twenty-minute class discussion led by me. As an experienced public speaker, I was looking forward to this. In each of the nine classes, I delivered a high-energy message about mindfulness, personal power, motivation, and success. I believed if any of my nine class lectures was made into a TEDx talk it would have gone viral; that's how good I felt about each one. Unfortunately, the students' demeanors told a different story. Few of the students paid attention to my lecture—and it had nothing to do with me. My energy was off the charts and my message was spot-on. If you saw the body language and facial expressions of these kids while I was talking, you would have thought I was dangling a pocket watch in front of them and swinging it back and forth. They looked like they were in a hypnotic trance. Many of them had their heads down and the majority looked like they hadn't slept in a week.

I went back to my office feeling a bit defeated. What was wrong with all of these kids? It's not like I hadn't done this before. I'd spoken to many classes over the years, and nothing had resembled this. Is this what teachers have to deal with every day? Then it hit me. The ninth graders I'd just spoken to were the "new" generation—the generation that received their first smartphones at earlier ages than those students just a couple of years ahead of them. These freshmen already had several years of smartphone addiction, social media dependency, and mental hijacking under their belts. And it showed. They were different. Their brains were different.

If you've ever seen an image of the human brain, you've likely noticed those electrical impulses that resemble tree branches extending from the outer wall of the brain. These tree branches are known as *neuropathways*, and they play an important role in human functionality. Each neuropathway influences how we communicate, cope, focus, concentrate, and socialize, just to name a few crucial functions. For example, if you've ever taken away your child's video game console or smartphone, the way they cope with this punishment has a lot to do with the development of their neuropathways. A child with healthy coping and emotional skills will naturally get a bit upset or be disappointed by the punishment, but a child with unhealthy coping and emotional skills might go into an uncontrolled fit of rage. And it seems that more and more children are displaying the latter.

· · · · ·

It takes a lot for a brain to change its wiring—typically three or more hours per day of consistent stimulating activity. Three hours per day might sound like a lot of stimulation, and it is. But according to a 2015 survey conducted by CNN, the typical thirteen-year-old spends a lot more than three hours per day engaged in highly stimulating brain activities.[5] Try eight or more hours per day, on average, seven days a week, spent staring at the bright lights of smartphones, tablets, and computer screens. The result: a new brain. A brain that is lit up like a Christmas tree; a brain that has literally grown new branches in order to adapt to the environment of cyberspace; a brain that is hyperfocused on tweets, snaps, and likes and not very focused on Mrs. Smith's classroom lectures or mine; a brain that is brilliant at communicating through texts and snaps but struggles with face-to-face communication. Those neuropathways have languished. Frightening!

A December 2015 study in the *Journal of Clinical Psychiatry* found that ADHD diagnoses have soared 43 percent in the United States in the first decade of this century, with more than one in ten youths now diagnosed with the disorder. The number of teenagers diagnosed with ADHD rose 52 percent between 2003 and 2015. And while ADHD is traditionally more common in boys than girls, the study also found a 55 percent increase in girls being diagnosed with the disorder.[6] This particular study was not designed to look for the underlying reasons for the changes, but it referred to past studies and suggested that the rise may be attributed to changing special education policy or increased public awareness. I disagree. I believe the increase in ADHD diagnoses has everything to do with the amount of time children are spending staring at screens.

A more recent study published in the *Journal of the American Medical Association* in July 2018 sought to determine whether the frequency of using digital media among fifteen- and sixteen-year-olds without significant ADHD symptoms was associated with subsequent occurrence of ADHD symptoms during a twenty-four-month follow-up. Among the 2,587 adolescents followed over this two-year period, there was a statistically significant but modest association between higher frequency of digital media use and subsequent symptoms of ADHD.[7]

CHANGING LANDSCAPES

When I first discovered this research into ADHD and neuroplasticity in 2009, I felt the need to educate parents, so I began lecturing. I called my lecture "Digitally Distracted: Parenting in the Age of Technology." While the bulk of my discussions involved brain neuroplasticity and ADHD symptoms, I also talked about how chronic video game playing, internet surfing, and television watching were affecting children in other ways. I included a lot of statistics that I'll discuss in the next chapter and warned parents that if they did not get a grip on their children's and their own media diets, we would see a surge in mental and emotional health disorders in the near future. Although the parents in attendance were fascinated by my lecture and told their friends about it, few took the necessary steps to change their children's media habits or their own. Looking back, I don't think they were ready for this groundbreaking information. After about two years of lecturing, I stopped. I became occupied with a television series I was hosting and focused on raising my own children. But I could not stop thinking about the problems that digital media was creating, problems that worsened as the next several years unfolded.

Around 2014 I felt the need to get out there and start speaking again. I couldn't sit on the sidelines anymore. I had to help parents and their children. It was my calling. So I began lecturing again locally. I'm glad I did, because now I speak all over the country at schools, parent groups, churches, and professional organizations. There is still a lot of work to be done, and I'm on a mission to do it.

The future problems that I predicted during my earlier lectures are now squarely upon us. More kids than ever before are emotionally fragile and lack critical coping skills because they are not spending enough time engaged in the real world, person to person. No matter where you go, whether it's the beach or a ball game, nearly everyone is disconnected from one another and connected to a handheld device instead. Our heads are buried in cyberspace, and face-to-face communication is slowly becoming a thing of the past. This lack of face-to-face interaction, particularly for children, reduces social and communication skills, making it difficult for them to handle the everyday bumps in the road of life. The end result: a substantial increase in stress, anxiety, and self-esteem issues, things I'm dealing with in record numbers.

Although my I&RS committee still receives referrals for students who are misdiagnosed with ADHD, over the last few years the pendulum has swung again. A whole new set of disabilities has emerged: anxiety disorders. Anxiety is now the number-one type of disability we deal with. And at my private counseling practice, I now receive more referrals for middle school children with major anxiety disorders over a one-year period than I used to receive in a ten-year period. At my high school I receive more calls from the nurse's office each week to help students who are having anxiety or panic issues than I used to receive in an entire school year. Do I think this has something to do with the amount of screen time these kids are immersed in? You better believe I do.

. . . . .

I want you to imagine the life of a typical sixteen-year-old girl for a moment. Let's call her Sarah. Sarah's mom enters her room each morning to wake her for school, because Sarah somehow slept through the buzz of her alarm clock even though it woke up the neighbors. Sarah didn't sleep much the night before because she couldn't pull herself away from the endless group chat she was a part of. After her mom's third or fourth attempt to wake her, Sarah finally emerges from her deep sleep. Her first instinct, before she has even realized she's awake, is to reach for her phone, which is on her nightstand within arm's reach. After she checks it, she yells at her mom and reluctantly gets on her feet. She proceeds to brush her teeth, change into her clothing, and eat breakfast as she catches up on the text messages and social media gossip left over from the night before. Finally, Sarah's mother is able to hurry her into the car in an effort to prevent her from being late to school. During the short commute, Sarah moves her thumbs vigorously across the screen of her smartphone, completely oblivious to the world around her, including her mom. By the time her mom has reached the drop-off point, Sarah has already sent and received dozens of text messages and snaps. As Sarah exits the car and walks toward the entrance of her school, her head is down, her eyes are fixated on her smartphone, and her thumbs are texting away. She never says thank you or goodbye to her mom. She is too distracted.

Unfortunately, this is an accurate portrayal of many modern-day kids. Because all of this has happened so quickly we struggle with ways to handle this behavior. We just don't know any better. For millions of boys and girls like Sarah around the world, this type of inappropriate behavior isn't just an occasional thing; it's an everyday thing. Most kids spend nearly every waking second of every day, seven days a week, glued to a screen, completely oblivious to life on earth. Their brains are disconnected from the world around them, making it difficult for them to handle real-life events and adversities. And it is starting earlier and earlier. The average age of first smartphone issuance is now 10.3 years old. This is crazy. It's way too young; there are too many risks. Let me illustrate.

You have a daughter who has just started middle school and you just bought her first smartphone. She is excited, but you have a few knots in your stomach. You set the ground rules, and everything is fine for the first couple of months. Your daughter is enjoying her device, and there aren't any hiccups except for having to tell her more than once that her time is up. But then things start to change rapidly; your daughter isn't the same. She's constantly staring into her phone, hypnotized by the glowing light. She's giving you an attitude all the time and seems addicted to the bright little box.

Then the problems start. As the months roll on you find yourself constantly having to tell her to get off of her phone, which always leads to an argument. Once an avid reader, your daughter rarely opens a book, and homework takes a back seat to everything else. Then the report card comes in and voila!—her grades have dropped. Once again an argument erupts, and you wonder what has happened to your wonderful, happy child. Your daughter is stressed all the time, and so are you. The tension in your home is unbearable, and you just don't know what to do. You want your life back.

Snapchat, Tiktoc, and Instagram enter her life. Soon they become her life. She spends hours every day posting pictures, checking for likes and follows, trying to keep up with it all. Every time you bring up your concerns she lashes out at you. You also notice that your daughter seems sad and often anxious. You wonder if it's just hormones. That might be part of it; after all, adolescence can be a difficult stage of development for many kids. Your child is changing biologically and emotionally. There is nothing easy about this developmental stage. Children are trying to figure out who they are, where they fit in, why they look weird, and what friend group they are a part of. But social media complicates this.

Social media adds another layer to the insecurity equation—a big layer. Your already insecure daughter now has a platform whereby she has constant access to all of her peers' perfect lives, a platform for comparing herself to others, a platform that provides an avalanche of shallow feedback in the form of likes and streaks. All of this, combined with adolescence, creates the perfect storm. Severe anxiety, insecurity, and even depression can start to surface. It is at this point when parents contact me at my private practice for help. The road ahead will be a long one.

In March 2018 Dr. Jean Twenge and I were invited to speak to a group of mental health professionals in Bend, Oregon. We gave separate lectures based on our research and experience about how screens and devices were impacting society. Dr. Twenge is a renowned research psychologist and professor at San Diego State University. She has conducted some of the most compelling studies so far about how screen time affects mental health. According to a 2017 study she led,

> Adolescents who spend more time on new media (including social media and electronic devices such as smartphones) were more likely to report mental health issues, while adolescents who spent more time on non screen activities (in-person social interaction, sports/exercise, homework, print media, and attending religious services) were less likely. Since 2010, IGen adolescents have spent more time on new media screen activities and less time on non screen activities, which may account for the increase in depression and suicide.[8]

Twenge also wrote an op-ed in March 2019 entitled, "The Mental Health Crisis among America's Youth Is Real—and It's Staggering." In it she says, "The first signs of a problem started to emerge around 2014: More young people said they felt overwhelmed and depressed. College counseling centers reported sharp increases in the number of students seeking treatment for mental health issues."[9] The article explains that although studies as far back as 2010 were showing increases in symptoms of depression and in suicide among adolescents, some researchers denied it. They felt it was overblown and that the data was insufficient. Those opinions have now been debunked. A 2017 study about mental health conducted by the US Department of Health and Human Services used a representative sample of the general population, not just those who sought help for mental health issues. Overall they surveyed over 600,000 Americans, and the study's results are indeed staggering. Here are some of the highlights:

- From 2009 to 2017, major depression among twenty- to twenty-one-year-olds more than doubled, rising from 7 percent to 15 percent.

- Depression surged 69 percent among sixteen- to seventeen-year-olds.

- Feelings of anxiety and hopelessness jumped 71 percent among eighteen- to twenty-five-year-olds from 2008 to 2017.

- Twice as many twenty-two- to twenty-three-year-olds attempted suicide in 2017 compared to 2008, and 55 percent more had suicidal thoughts.[10]

What changed? Could it be that smartphones started to become mainstream right around 2008? That would mean that the twenty-two- and twenty-three-year-olds mentioned in the study were thirteen or fourteen in 2008, and most likely had gotten their first smartphone and started using social media.

The study also found that by 2017, one out of five twelve- to seventeen-year-old girls had experienced major depression the previous year, and that the suicide rate among eighteen- to nineteen-year-olds climbed 56 percent from 2008 to 2017. Because suicide is at a fifty-year peak, the average US life expectancy has gone down. The significant changes found in the study are almost exclusively among teens and young adults, with very little change among people over the age of twenty-six.

Does that sound fatalistic? Let me assure you, I believe that many of the mental health issues I'm seeing are preventable. If parents could simply delay the age that they give their children smartphones and allow them to use social media, we would see different statistics. Many parents I meet around the country tell me that the biggest mistake they made was getting their child a smartphone. I've never had one parent come up to me after a lecture or email me to tell me that getting their child a smartphone was the smartest or best thing they ever did for their child.

We all know it's a bad idea to hand an eleven- or twelve-year-old a smartphone—but we do it. We give in to the pressure. We fear that our child will be isolated or left out if he or she is the only one without a phone. I get it! In fact, I'm living it! My daughter is a sixth grader and is one of only a few children in her grade without a phone. She pleads with me every day to get her one, and I say no. Call me a bad dad; that's ok. If I were to get her a phone I would be the world's biggest hypocrite. All we have to do is delay the age at which our children get these digital weapons of mass destruction or ensure they don't have any social media, and we wouldn't be having this conversation about the mental health and suicide crisis ripping through our society.

NEURAL PRUNING

Earlier in the chapter I talked about neuroplasticity, which is the brain's way of reorganizing itself and creating new connections. Although it can have negative consequences, something else called *neural pruning* is even more concerning. Neural pruning is a natural and normal occurrence during adolescence; it's the brain's way of weeding out pathways that are used less often. If you've seen the movie *Inside Out* you'll recognize neural pruning as the process that occurs as eleven-year-old Riley tries to assimilate her family's move to a new city. Joy and the other emotions inside her brain fight against this neural pruning but finally accept it as part of the maturing process. But these changes in the brain aren't always positive. For example, if young folks spend more time communicating through a smartphone than they do face-to-face, the brain will weed out the neural pathways that are necessary for becoming good face-to-face communicators.

Although more research needs to be done about neural pruning, it might explain why a lot of young adults are struggling with simple skills like having a conversation with a stranger or interviewing for a job. A lot of my friends and colleagues in management positions often interview folks fresh out of college. They tell me that many of these job candidates are missing something. On paper they look great but in person they lack oomph and have poor communication skills. Sitting through a face-to-face interview seems unnatural to them. I also experience this at my private counseling practice. Many of the teens I counsel have a hard time making eye contact or seem a little bit more anxious than usual. A lot of my jokes seem to go right over their heads too. More parents than ever tell me that their children struggle to form friendships and are rarely invited to friends' homes or have friends over at their home. Could this growing crop of social and communication problems be the result of neural pruning? Maybe! Ask yourself this question: If the neuropathways that are responsible for producing strong social and communication skills have been compromised, how is it possible to be, well, social?

Another issue I'm dealing with more regularly is poor coping skills. Over the last several years there have been an unprecedented number of meltdowns in my office from students who have received a low grade on a test or experienced a mean comment on social media. Could this have something to do with neural pruning too? I think so. The bottom line is this: more kids than ever before are struggling to communicate, socialize, or cope effectively with real-life matters because they are not living in the real world. I believe a short-circuiting effect has occurred in their brains, sending their emotions into a tailspin and creating a host of different mental and emotional disorders.

· · · · ·

When I was a graduate student in the late 1990s, I took a course called "The Biopsychosocial Perspectives of Drugs." The professor, Dr. Hamaerle, told us the following story about how addiction can change brain functionality.

One night a forty-five-year-old man was pulled over by a police officer for having a broken taillight. When he rolled down the window and handed the officer his license and registration, the officer noticed an overwhelming smell of alcohol coming from his car and asked him if he had been drinking. The man responded that he had not. Although the man wasn't slurring his words and showed no signs of intoxication, the officer asked him to step out of the car because he couldn't get past the strong smell of alcohol. The officer conducted the appropriate field sobriety tests, which the man passed with flying colors. He showed no signs of intoxication whatsoever. The officer still could not dismiss the smell of alcohol permeating the air, so he brought the man to the station to conduct a Breathalyzer exam just to be certain.

At the time, the legal blood alcohol content (BAC) was .10 and anyone with a .10 or higher would be charged with a DWI. Keep in mind that for an average person a BAC of .20 would render them extremely intoxicated, a .30 would likely result in a coma, and a .40 would usually mean death.

This man's BAC reading was .62. Astounding!

How is it that this man was even alive, let alone showing no signs of intoxication? The following day, when the man was sober, he was released from his jail cell; it was then that he started displaying the classic signs of intoxication, including slurred speech, body tremors, and an inability to walk straight.

This story demonstrates the power of the human brain. Since the man was a seasoned alcoholic who drank excessively every day, his brain adapted to its new normal—being intoxicated. Sobriety was foreign to his brain and intoxication was normal. The story of the alcoholic is similar to my experiences with a lot of the children and teenagers I counsel. Because cyberspace is where they spend most of their time, the real world is a foreign place. Unfortunately when some of these youngsters reach adulthood they will end up like a former client of mine, whom I'll call Jan.[11]

Jan was a twenty-four-year-old millennial I began seeing at my private counseling practice to help her with anxiety. I could feel her anxiety the moment I met her, before she even said a word. She was an emotional wreck. Jan told me that she was always anxious and could not figure out how to get rid of this constant, uncomfortable feeling. She needed help. Although she was a college graduate, she worked part-time in a non-challenging job because it was safe for her; her anxiety prevented her from going out into the world and pursuing the kind of career her college degree would allow. As I got to know Jan I started to explore her screen time. I asked her to describe for me her normal routine when she got home from work each evening. She said that she would typically log on to her computer, scroll around on her smartphone, and watch television. I gave her a two-part daily assignment that I wanted her to try between sessions. First, I asked her to track her feelings when she was using an electronic device to see if she felt any anxiety during those times. Next, I asked her to sit in total silence every day for fifteen minutes, without any distractions getting in the way, including electronic devices. She explained to me that she had never done anything like this before but agreed to give it a try.

When Jan returned the following week she told me that she did not experience any anxiety while using her electronic devices, which is what I had expected. During her fifteen-minute meditations, however, while she was disconnected from electronics, she experienced extreme panic and anxiety and was only able to do the assignment twice. I concluded that because Jan was constantly connected to the cyber-world, the real world had turned into a frightening, foreign place for her. Look at it like this: What would happen to a lion if it were released into the wild after having lived its entire life in a cage? The lion would not survive because its natural habitat would now be the cage, not the wilderness.

The wilderness would seem foreign to the lion. Jan was no different. She functioned just fine in her cyberworld but not in her real world. It would take a lot of work to get her brain to readapt to the real world.

UNNATURAL HABITAT

Many of the younger people I counsel are future Jans. As I mentioned earlier, not a day goes by that I'm not calming down a high school student having an emotional breakdown over something trivial. Later we'll discuss what it takes for children to strengthen their emotional intelligence and how we can help them. But for now I will leave you with a few examples of some teenagers I counseled in the days just before writing this chapter.

One day I received a phone call from a distressed parent whose teenage son needed to be assessed for suicidal ideation before he could return to school. Luckily, I was able to get the family in for an appointment that night. They seemed like a very well-rounded family, yet the boy was emotionally distraught. Here is what transpired: the boy's father found inappropriate content on the boy's phone and took it away from him as a punishment. The next morning, the parents found a lengthy note from the boy that resembled a suicide note. The boy felt that he could not go on living without his phone as he would "have no life" and no friends. That night, they were in my office.

The next day, I received a call from a very concerned mom about her daughter, who'd had an emotional breakdown because she discovered on social media that her best friend was getting together with another girl; she was afraid her best friend was going to drop her. As my conversation progressed with the mother, she told me she had read some material her daughter had secretly written. The girl expressed that she felt unpopular, ugly, and uncomfortable around people and that she wished she would die. When I asked the mom about her daughter's social media use, the mom told me that her daughter was on social media and her smartphone 24/7.

Then a coach friend of mine told me a story about something that had happened to her over the weekend. Her team had taken an overnight trip to Connecticut, and the owner of the facility where they stayed and played their games had a rule: no cell phones allowed during the entire trip. The owner felt that they were a distraction to the players and affected team camaraderie. A parent of one of the players threatened to sue the owner because he felt his rights were violated—he couldn't contact his daughter on her phone in the event of an emergency. I wonder if this man's daughter struggles with fear and worry.

I want to make one thing clear: I do not think an hour or two of screen time each day is bad. But eight hours per day is. Look at it like this: if you exercised for an hour or two every day that would be a good thing; if you worked out hard for eight or nine hours a day that wouldn't be.

Before we move on to the next chapter, I want to share one last story. Four years ago I accompanied my nine-year-old daughter's class on a field trip to a raptor hospital. The instructor showed the class a beautiful barn owl that had been injured when it was young. The barn owl had lived at the facility for a number of years and was very accustomed to humans. The children loved it. One of the children asked the facilitator why the owl had not been released back into the wild. The facilitator explained that although the owl's injury had healed, the owl would die if it were released into the wild because it would not know how to hunt for prey and would therefore starve. Essentially, the owl would not know how to survive in its natural habitat.

Our children aren't much different from that barn owl. No, their electronic devices aren't going to kill them, but they have the capacity to inhibit them greatly. We need to make sure that our children are developing in their natural habitat, the physical world around them, not the cyberworld. Children are meant to be playing outside with other children, getting dirty, and scraping their knees. Their imaginations beg them to look up at the sky and make shapes out of clouds. That is what they were born to do. So let's make sure they spend less time indoors staring at screens and more time outdoors staring at the sky.

CHAPTER TIPS

1. The American Association of Pediatrics recommends no more than two hours per day of total screen time for entertainment purposes for children over age eight. Stick to this recommendation and many of the scary things I explained in this chapter will likely never occur.

2. Delay the age at which you purchase a smartphone for your child to at least late adolescence. The longer you wait, the better off you and your child will be. Don't worry about what other families are allowing. This is your family; play by your rules, not theirs.

3. If your child already has a smartphone and seems immersed in it, it's not too late to make some changes. Chapter 3 starts off with a great example.

4. If your child is suffering from anxiety or depression, get them help immediately.

CHAPTER 2

Cyberspace Children

A Full-Time Job

In 2005 the Kaiser Family Foundation released the findings from a 2004 study on children's media use. The study tracked trends in the amount and types of electronic media that kids used. Their findings revealed that the average eight- to eighteen-year-old spent six hours and thirty minutes per day using electronic media.[1] The researchers intended to conduct the study every four years, but when 2008 came around they were hesitant because they felt the numbers had to have a ceiling. They didn't think it was possible for kids to spend more time using electronic media than the previous study had revealed. There just weren't enough hours in the day for the number to increase. They conducted the study again anyway—and were stunned by the outcome. The amount of time children were using electronic media had risen by over an hour to seven hours and thirty-eight minutes per day, seven days a week.[2] The average kid in America was spending more time each week plugged in to electronic devices than the average full-time worker was spending at work. In fact, kids were spending more time using electronic devices than they spent on any other activity including sleep.

There were two things that occurred between 2004 and 2008 that led to this increase: YouTube and Facebook were born.

The 2008 Kaiser study tracked four specific types of media: television, computers, video games, and music devices.

TELEVISION

- The average eight- to eighteen-year-old spent four-and-a-half hours per day watching TV.
- 99 percent of households had at least one television.
- 80 percent of homes had three televisions.
- 71 percent of all eight- to eighteen-year-olds had a television in their bedroom; these kids spent an hour more per day watching television.
- 50 percent of eleven- to fourteen-year-olds had no television-watching rules.
- 75 percent of fifteen- to eighteen-year-olds had no television-watching rules.
- 64 percent of households left the television on during dinner.
- By age eighteen, the average adolescent will have seen 200,000 acts of violence on television.

COMPUTERS

- The amount of time spent using computers increased by 50 percent from 2004 to 2008.
- The three most popular computer activities were social networking sites, computer games, and YouTube.

- 62 percent of kids claimed that they lied to their parents about what they looked at on the web.
- 53 percent deleted their browsing history so parents couldn't discover what they'd been up to.
- 75 percent of seventh to twelfth graders had created a profile on a social media site.
- The average eleven- to fourteen-year-old spent one hour and seven minutes per day on Facebook.

VIDEO GAMES

- 50 percent of kids had a video game system in their bedroom.
- 52 percent of all video games were played on handheld devices.
- Those who did play video games spent two hours a day doing so.
- 25 percent of eight- to ten-year-olds played violent video games.
- 60 percent of eleven- to fourteen-year-olds played violent video games.
- 72 percent of fifteen- to eighteen-year-olds played violent video games.

MUSIC DEVICES

- Listening to music was the second most popular media activity among eight- to eighteen-year-olds.
- Eight- to ten-year-olds spent one hour and eight minutes per day listening to music.
- Eleven- to fourteen-year-olds spent two hours and twenty-two minutes per day listening to music.

- Fifteen- to eighteen-year-olds spent three hours and three minutes per day listening to music.

The 2008 Kaiser study also concluded that by age twenty-one, each member of this generation will have:

- Played more than 10,000 hours of video games.
- Sent and received 250,000 emails and texts.
- Spent 10,000 hours on phones.
- Watched more than 20,000 hours of TV.
- Seen more than 500,000 commercials.[3]

Although these statistics are alarming, there's something even more alarming: *the Kaiser study did not include smartphone or tablet use* because they weren't relevant in 2008. Today, no matter where you go, the majority of people are walking around with a smartphone in hand, a device that fits in our palm and gives us access to every form of media, television, gaming, music, social media, and the internet. If kids in 2008 were spending seven hours and thirty-eight minutes per day using electronic media when they didn't even have smartphones yet, how much time are they spending now?

In October 2015, Common Sense Media conducted a large-scale, probability-based survey to explore young people's media diets. These more up-to-date findings showed that the average American teenager spent nine hours per day, or sixty-three hours per week, immersed in electronic media, not including school-related technology. Individuals in the study who were labeled "heavy" users spent an incredible thirteen hours and twenty minutes a day with screen media.[4]

PHYSICAL REALITIES

Remember Sarah, the teenager who was glued to her smartphone the moment she got out of bed? If you were to take a stroll through the hallways of your local high school while kids were switching classes, you would be shocked by the scene. Nearly every student is walking the halls with their head and neck down, headphones in their ears, and eyes fixated on a device. If you made your way over to the cafeteria during a lunch period you'd notice most students staring into a laptop, tablet, or phone, disconnected from one another. Make your way over to the homes of these kids and the picture would be just as bleak: very little interaction between family members and plenty of interaction with invisible friends on the receiving end of each text and post. And it goes way beyond our schools and homes.

Screen addiction has gotten so ubiquitous that it is causing deaths and injuries. We hear about these stories all the time, from texting pedestrians being struck by cars to daredevils taking selfies as they hang from the roofs of buildings. It's out of control. According to a July 14, 2016, article in the *LA Times*, two men fell off the edge of an ocean bluff and had to be rescued by firefighters because they were playing the game Pokemon Go, and another player was stabbed in a park in a separate incident.[5] These are just a couple of examples of many reported by police across the nation shortly after the game was released.

When so much energy is funneled into such diversions, there's none left for basic human functions. A January 2016 headline in the *New York Post* proclaimed, "Many NYC Students So Tech-Oriented They Can't Even Sign Their Own Names." That's right, scores of students in New York City, including the children of some state lawmakers, can't sign their own names because all they know are keypads and screens.[6] Not only is screen addiction reducing our children's mental and emotional capacity, and causing injuries and deaths, but it's also affecting our children's fine motor skills. Yes, this is pretty scary, but I'm not done yet!

Studies conducted with college students over the past few years have found that smartphones are making most of them hallucinate. That's right—hallucinate. It is called "phantom vibration syndrome." Roughly once every two weeks, the majority of the students who were surveyed experienced a "phantom vibration," or a buzzing sensation in their pocket, even though their phone wasn't vibrating. According to Robert Rosenberger, a professor in the School of Public Policy at Georgia Tech, "The phone actually becomes a part of you, and you become trained to perceive the phone's vibrations as an incoming call or text. When a phone shifts in the pocket, it triggers a muscle spasm in your leg that resembles a phone vibration, even though no one is calling."[7]

About eighteen years ago, after I bought my first cell phone, I experienced this phenomenon. I always kept my cell phone in my pocket on vibrate, and occasionally I felt it vibrate only to reach into my empty pocket and discover that my phone was on my desk. At first I didn't realize why I was having this sensation and figured it must be a kind of Pavlovian reaction. I even went to a doctor just to make sure there wasn't something wrong with me. I remember asking the doctor if it was possible that the muscles in my leg had learned to experience the vibration from my phone. He paused with a puzzled look on his face, then admitted, "Yes, I guess that is possible." I think I taught that doctor something that day.

Other research suggests that "selfies" can be dangerous to your health. I'm not referring to the stories of people falling off cliffs or walking into traffic; I'm talking about legitimate physical health issues. Helena Horton, a journalist writing for the UK newspaper *The Telegraph*, has documented a phenomenon called "selfie stomach" experienced by many internet and selfie addicts.[8] Horton referred in particular to a twenty-one-year-old self-proclaimed "selfie addict" named Michelle Gore who contracted a painful condition known as Tietze disease from taking too many selfies. The disorder is caused by putting too much strain on your rib cartilage from sucking in your gut. Gore was taking approximately two hundred selfies per day and even had a waterproof case for her phone so that she could stay connected while in the shower. Gore finally decided to unplug after she woke one morning to find herself tangled up in cables from all of her different gadgets.

Another physical abnormality occurring in younger generations is something dubbed "tech neck." If you haven't heard of this condition, picture the sagging skin under the chins and jaws of older people. This latest ailment can be found in people between eighteen and thirty-nine years old, and dermatologists blame smartphones and tablets because of the repeated bending of the neck to look at portable device screens. This sagging of the jowls used to be found only in people in their late middle age, but now a lot of younger people are visiting dermatologists for the condition.[9]

Back and neck problems are another concern. A study in *Surgery Technology International* found that heavy portable device use causes back and neck problems.

As the head tilts forward the forces seen by the neck surges to 27 pounds at 15 degrees, 40 pounds at 30 degrees, 49 pounds at 45 degrees and 60 pounds at 60 degrees. [Chronic screen staring could] deteriorate the back and neck muscles to the point of needing surgery.[10]

By far the most frightening health effect from handheld devices and gadgets is cancer. Even though the wireless industry does not want you to know it, just a little bit of cell phone use can cause a big increase in brain cancer risk. To understand this risk, first you need to understand that cell phones—all of them—emit radio frequency (RF) radiation. The effects of our exposure to this are just starting to be understood. Researchers at the Yale School of Medicine and renowned physician Dr. Devra Davis claim that cell phones do in fact cause brain cancer. At a symposium in May 2016, the Yale researchers and Dr. Davis presented several reports maintaining that the developing brains of young children absorb twice the amount of radiation as adult brains do. Doctors at the symposium feared that prolonged exposure to radiation during childhood would cause cancer later in life. Researchers say it will be a long time before they know how risky cell phone use really is, because cancers like brain tumors take ten to twenty years to take root. Doctors at the symposium also warned that the infant brain, even in the womb, is particularly vulnerable to cell phone radiation. Dr. Davis advises pregnant women to keep the phone away from the abdomen, particularly toward the end of pregnancy.[11]

If it's so dangerous, you might ask, why haven't you heard anything about it until now? In March 2017 the *San Francisco Chronicle* published an article entitled, "State Kept Secret Guidelines on Safe Cellphone Use," which reported that for years state health officials kept secret a set of guidelines meant to inform the public about the risks associated with cell phone use and the best practices to avoid potential harm.[12] Joel Moskowitz, a public health researcher at UC Berkeley, had to sue the California public department of health in order to have these guidelines released. The whole process took years. Moskowitz believes that lives could have been saved if the guidelines had been published by the department when the results came out seven years earlier. He believes politics and industry interference are to blame. Thankfully a Sacramento superior court judge, Sheelyanne Chang, ordered for the release of the guidelines in February 2017. The two-page guidelines are based on studies that suggest increases in brain cancer and other health problems from long-term cell phone use.[13]

Chang said she found it "pretty astounding" that a public health department would argue that it shouldn't have to release such important findings gathered by its own scientists. I remember feeling very excited when I found out about the guidelines being released to the public. I thought for sure it would be headline news, but I was wrong. The media released the guidelines with very little urgency. Few people ever learned about them. I suppose the mainstream media didn't think this information was important, or perhaps they are in cahoots with Big Tech. To date, not many people are aware of these guidelines or the dangers of cell phone radiation, and the cellular industry wouldn't have it any other way.

The *San Francisco Chronicle* article also explains that cell phones carry warnings buried in the settings of the phone where most people would never look. Dr. Davis has a website called showthefingerprint.org, which helps users find these warnings and encourages manufacturers to put the information where users can find it. The wireless industry strongly opposes this—of course! In fact the wireless communication industry has an organization that strong-arms their opposition. It's called CTIA, and it spends over $11 million a year lobbying for them. CTIA went as far as seeking a court order to ban the disclosure of those cell phone guidelines I mentioned. They claimed there wasn't enough evidence and that experts showed no health risks from the radiation emitted from cell phones, even though there were more than ten peer-reviewed studies showing an increased risk in brain tumors along with other health ailments. On its website, CTIA promises, "5G will be transformative—making our lives better, our communities safer and our nation more prosperous."[14] No caveats in sight.

Before we talk about 5G, I want to discuss another large-scale study conducted by the National Institute of Health's National Toxicology Program. In April 2018 an expert peer-review panel found that RF radiation showed a definitive link to heart and brain tumors in rats. Thousands of rats that were exposed to radiation emitted by smartphones for nine hours a day showed "clear evidence of carcinogenicity."[15] The radiation also caused a significant increase in cancers of the liver, prostate, pancreas, and more. According to Dr. Davis, "Studies of people with 10 or more years of exposure to cell phones show higher risks for tumors." She "warns of 'increasing exposures' in schools and homes throughout the nation, and points out the folly of children being routinely given 'two-way microwave radiating devices to use next to their developing bodies.'"[16] Also, despite all of the research regarding the dangers of 5G exposure, "CTIA [predictably] maintains that an already existing body of peer-reviewed studies shows that there are no established health effects from RF radiation from cell phones."[17]

Now back to 5G and CTIA's comments on their website; 5G is spreading all over the world, and it's a lot more powerful than 4G. We are the human test subjects. As reported in a June 2017 article on *NaturalHealth365*, "Smart Cities" are starting to pop up. These are cities that will include 5G wireless antennas on most utility poles and internet sensors everywhere. The exposure to radiation will increase dramatically. Unfortunately, most people will be oblivious to the dangers of 5G and the increase in electromagnetic frequency (EMF) pollution.[18]

Your current smartphone runs on 4G or 3G technology, which utilizes a limited range of the microwave spectrum. According to the article, 5G, which stands for "5th generation," will greatly expand the amount of spectrum used and include higher gigahertz range frequencies never used before on devices. These frequencies are extremely powerful. When 5G takes over, we'll be able to download a movie in seconds. This may sound amazing, but it comes with the potential for extreme danger. Because the 5G frequency doesn't travel as far as 4G, antennas will need to be placed on most utility poles in your neighborhood, my neighborhood, and any neighborhood that boasts 5G access. That's millions of antennas. This will essentially blanket all of us in microwave radiation, creating an electromagnetic environment never seen before. Sadly, you probably know nothing about this, and you're certainly not going to find it on CTIA's website.

The *NaturalHealth365* article goes on to explain that our current laws make the rollout of the 5G network difficult for wireless companies. Of course the wireless industry is pressing for weaker regulations, and Senator John Thune of South Dakota, for example, is listening. He introduced a bill, SB 19, called the *Mobil Now Act* that would weaken those regulations and take away communities' ability to regulate the placement of these cellular antennas. Wireless companies would be able to put the antennas right outside your bedroom window, and you wouldn't be able to do a thing about it. I'd like to know how much "donation money" Senator Thune's campaign receives from the wireless industry. The only way around this is to call your senators today and put some pressure on them.

"This technology will also make its way into our homes and fill them with appliances and devices that pulse microwave radiation."[19] These "smart homes" include appliances, thermostats, and security systems, for example, that can be controlled wirelessly. Unfortunately this will expand the amount of EMF pollution in our homes as these items "pulse hundreds of thousands of times each day, greatly expanding the amount of EMF pollution in homes."[20] The biggest pot of gold for the tech industry will come from the "immense personal data" they will be able to collect from us.[21] This is worth billions to marketers while it destroys our personal privacy.

School may no longer be safe either. A March 2019 article on a local CBS website in Sacramento reported that parents blamed the radiation emitting from San Joaquin Elementary School's cell tower after four students at the school were diagnosed with cancer.[22] The school district had tests done on the tower and claims that it meets federal regulations, but parents in the community aren't buying it and are hiring their own experts. Eric Winheim, an electromagnetic radiation specialist interviewed for the article, says, "I wouldn't send my kids there at all, it absolutely is dangerous. Children are still developing and their cells are still being divided. It's the worst possible time in their life to be exposed."[23] Winheim explains that it's more than just a tower; it transmits wireless frequencies. Parents want the tower removed but claim the school district won't budge because it receives $2,000 a month to house the tower.

. . . . .

If organizations in the States won't budge, we'll have to look elsewhere for leadership in this oncoming health crisis. Perhaps Belgium will be the global leader that paves the way toward better regulations and a greater understanding of the dangerous consequences of 5G. According to an April 2019 article written by Josh del Sol Beaulieu, a Belgian government minister named Céline Fremault announced that Brussels is halting its 5G plans due to health effects. Fremault says, "I cannot welcome such technology if the radiation standards, which must protect the citizen, are not respected, 5G or not. The people of Brussels are not guinea pigs whose health I can sell at a profit. We cannot leave anything to doubt."[24]

Beaulieu claims that 5G pushback is starting to go viral as there is a compilation of videos about the dangers of 5G and the shocking state of greed among the agenda pushers. He says,

When the industry sheep are being presented with an avalanche of scientific evidence for a catastrophe-in-the-making, and yet they refuse to listen and instead continue to tow [sic] the profit-pushing line, what becomes visible is the *shadow-expression of utter disdain for life.* That may sound harsh, but I encourage you to consider this deeply.[25]

Beaulieu calls this a type of hive-mind syndrome. The agenda pushers are "so frenzied with dollar-signs" that they are "incapable of self-corrective thought," even though all of this is obviously heading for them and their own kids too. Money and greed come before our health. The cronyism is so bad that "the talking heads of the wireless industry even brashly admit—when forced, in a US Senate hearing—that they had not done any safety studies . . . and they don't plan to."[26]

I know this all sounds scary, and it is. But it isn't hopeless. There are steps you can take to protect your children and yourself.

- Discontinue use of air pods and other types of Bluetooth headsets as they emit powerful microwaves—right next to the brain. Do not allow your children to use air pods. My son was given a pair as a gift and he is not allowed to use them.
- Never put your phone near your head and advise your children to do the same. Use the speakerphone or wired headphones for calls.
- Unless your phone is on airplane mode, keep it out of your pockets and away from your bra straps. Make sure your children do the same.
- Try to move toward wired technology, like Ethernet and fiber optics.
- Turn your wireless router off at night. It emits radiation throughout your entire home.

- Stay away from wireless baby monitors.
- Form a group in your community with other parents and demand that the school your children attend uses wired technology instead of wireless.

DISTRACTIBILITY

The potential long-term health effects of our hyperconnected world are alarming, but I know that for many of us, the short-term effects are causing mayhem in the here and now. I recently attended a meeting with some administrators and teachers at my school with regard to some of the student issues we are dealing with. Everyone agreed that the biggest challenge we face is dealing with the declining mental health of our students. During our meeting everything we discussed about student academics and mental health problems circled back to screen time. The principal spoke of how, on several occasions, when he greeted students in the hallway they ignored him. He found this to be quite rude until he realized that they weren't actually ignoring him—they were just too distracted by the music playing in their headphones to notice him. A lot of kids have a pair over their ears at all times.

Next, the vice principal spoke of an article he read in the local paper about a twenty-seven-year-old man who was tragically killed by a train. The railroad tracks where the man was killed are in Ramsey, New Jersey, close to where I live. There are two sets of tracks parallel to each other at the intersection. When a commuter train stops at the tracks, the gate goes down and it is impossible to see another train coming on the set of parallel tracks. This isn't the first time someone has been killed at this railroad stop. Several years ago, a man was waiting at the intersection while the gate was down and the train was fully stopped. He decided to walk around the front of the stopped train, forgetting that a train could be coming on the other set of tracks. Unfortunately, another commuter train was traveling down those tracks and killed the man instantly. After this tragic event the railroad company plastered warning signs all over the intersection.

The more recent story shared by my vice principal was similar except for one thing: the young man was wearing headphones. I don't believe the headphones prevented him from hearing the other train, because the parked train itself is quite loud. It would be impossible for the average person not to hear the whistle of the other train. I believe this young man was distracted by his headphones and failed to notice the great big warning signs plastered all over the place.

Many children in our schools, especially in high schools, have earbuds in their ears as they walk the halls and eat their lunch. They are in their own little world and often oblivious to what's going on around them. They won't be hit by a train in the hallway, but they will lose important social skills and fail to notice all of the wonderful things happening in the world around them.

For many kids, this distraction is available around the clock. A lot of parents I work with allow their children to listen to music while doing their homework because their kids tell them it helps them focus better. Although more research needs to be done, I don't think playing loud music helps a child solve difficult math equations or write effective English essays, because it distracts the brain. If you disagree, try it for yourself. The next time you are reading a novel, listen to your favorite music at the same time. You will find this to be very difficult. I read all the time while I am exercising on the elliptical machine, and whenever a song I like is played over the gym's speakers, I find it impossible to retain what I've just read. A lot of kids have become so used to wearing headphones or earbuds all the time that they feel uncomfortable when not wearing them. Truly focusing on anything else—a book, a lecture, a set of instructions—might constitute an uncomfortable experience for these kids.

But whose behavior really paved the way for this era of distractibility? It's not just our kids who are constantly distracted by screens; so are adults. A couple of years ago I was driving my son and two of his friends home from a Boy Scout camping trip. One of the roads home was a four-lane roadway in each direction with a lot of traffic lights along the way. We approached a traffic light that had just turned red, and I was the second car in line in my lane; all four lanes were occupied. I said to the boys, "How much do you want to bet that when the light turns green one of those four cars in the first row won't move because the driver is looking at their phone?" I also predicted that other drivers would start beeping their horns to get the person's attention. Well, I was wrong. When the light turned green, not just one of the four cars failed to move but rather two. After about three seconds the horns started blaring. The boys were amazed.

After that experience I decided to conduct an informal survey to see how many drivers looked at their phones while stopped at red lights. I found several traffic lights near my house that had an area where I could park my car and get a good look into cars stopped at the red light. It was a little more difficult than I thought it would be, but over the course of several weeks, I surveyed over three hundred drivers. A little more than 50 percent of drivers checked their phones when stopped at a red light. Many of them continued to glance up and down as they drove off after the light turned green.

The purpose of my survey wasn't about the dangers of texting and driving but more about the obsessive need to look at a screen every spare second we have, including while stuck at a red light. I fear what is going to happen to our tech-obsessed kids when they get their driver's licenses!

How obsessed are we? You've heard those stories about people walking into lampposts and fountains and so on. I read one recently about a woman who crashed her car because she was watching a Netflix movie on her tablet while driving. Seriously? Did you know that the pedestrian death rate by automobile has skyrocketed in recent years from the combination of distracted walkers and distracted drivers? Unbelievable! And just when you think you've heard it all, now there's texting while breastfeeding, also known as "brexting."

Brexting has become a common trend for young, nursing moms because many of them established their social media habits before parenthood. In an article written on Southern California Public Radio's website, experts say this trend is becoming more and more common and has caused debates about whether or not it is ok to be on the phone while breastfeeding. The experts sourced in the article caution against extended smartphone use during breastfeeding or bottle-feeding as it can affect the important bonding time between mother and child. Terry Bretscher, a nurse and lactation supervisor, explains, "It is very hard to bond and talk to the baby if you are on the phone."[27] Bretscher sees this firsthand; she and her staff try to discourage new moms from this practice. The article explains that moms who brext will miss important messages from their baby and inhibit the secure attachment that is important during feeding. One thing not mentioned in the article is the radiation exposure. Remember, an infant's brain absorbs double the amount of radiation as an adult brain. The phone can't get any closer to an infant's brain than while nursing or bottle-feeding.

The evidence is clear: we are screen-obsessed, and this obsession affects our children and us in both the long term and short term—and not just physically.

CHAPTER TIPS

1. Keep all screens out of your child's bedroom.
2. Be a role model. Adults are spending just as much time in front of screens as kids. We must practice what we preach, and that means powering off our own devices more often when we are with our children.
3. If your child already has a phone, send your child to school without it.
4. If you are a new mom, never feed your baby and use a device simultaneously.
5. Contact your local elected officials and demand that they ban 5G from your neighborhood.

CHAPTER 3

Social Media and the Development of Self-Esteem

Twelve-year-old Abby Jones is already changing the world with her efforts in philanthropy and her "pay it forward" mentality. She believes that the key to success comes down to having open, honest, and caring relationships with one another. Abby also has an important message for parents who are struggling with their children's screen time and social media addictions. In December 2018, Abby delivered a powerful, slap-in-the-face TEDx talk to over five hundred adults. I found out about it from her mom, who had reached out to me to let me know that her daughter read the first edition of this book, and it changed her life and inspired her to give the TEDx talk. After watching the talk on YouTube, I got chills down my spine and immediately contacted a producer I knew from *The Today Show* to share Abby's story with her. The following week NBC flew Abby and her mom to their studios in New York, where the three of us talked about Abby's story live on *The Today Show*. It was such a pleasure to meet Abby and her mom and to help spread her important message even further.

Abby's TEDx talk is called, "From 'I Hate You' to 'Thank You.'"[1] It's just under ten minutes long and is a must-watch. A smart, witty twelve-year-old steps onto a stage for the first time in front of hundreds of adults and delivers the bomb. She told me in NBC's green room that she was incredibly nervous before her talk but did it anyway because she felt it was so important. Here's her story: a few months prior to her TEDx talk, Abby downloaded Instagram on her phone. Immediately mesmerized by it, she began spending hours and hours on it trying to get more followers, views, and likes. She became so focused on getting more "likes" on her posts and views on her "stories" that she completely lost interest in what was going on around her. Her real life disappeared and was replaced by the fake life of Instagram.

And then her phone, "her everything," was taken away for a whole month after her mom discovered a post that she did not approve of. In her talk Abby explains that during the first week without her phone she became very angry with her parents. She feared that everyone at her school was going to judge her and notice that she didn't have a phone. She thought she would have no source of entertainment because everyone else around her was always on their phones and didn't talk to her. And she no longer carried a book with her, even though, until recently, she'd always had her nose in a book. She would have nothing to do. It was at this point that Abby said "I hate you" to her parents.

During Abby's second week without her phone, she started to realize that no one really noticed she didn't have it. No one judged her. By week three she began to realize that not having a phone was for her own good, as she could now see how it had negatively impacted her. Her friends and family told her that they liked being around her more because she behaved better and communicated better without her phone. Abby realized that life without a phone was a better life for her.

By the fourth week Abby felt free. She could go outside and play Frisbee with her dad and play with her friends without feeling the vibration from her phone every two seconds. It felt like a burden had been lifted from her shoulders. She was no longer a slave to her phone. It was at this point that she picked up a book again, the first edition of the book you are presently reading. Her mom had purchased it and left it on the kitchen counter. Abby couldn't put it down because the message spoke directly to her. It was at this point that she said "thank you" to her parents. Abby is now inspiring other children around the world to spend less time on screens and more time in person. She tells parents that they need to start being parents again to their children, not friends. And sometimes that means taking away the things that they will be the most angry about, because those are often the most stressful and problematic things in their life. Thank you, Abby!

．．．．．

Neuroplasticity, the brain's ability to adapt to its environment by rewiring its circuitry, may be connected to mental and emotional health issues, but what is the actual content children are exposed to through social media, and how can it impact them emotionally? I'm not talking about extreme examples we hear about but rather the innocuous, innocent stuff shared 24/7 on sites like Snapchat and Twitter.

These types of posts might seem harmless when compared to overtly violent or sexual posts, but there is more than meets the eye. Let me explain.

As posts, pictures, and texts continue their endless flow between our children and others, they can pose unforeseen problems. Take, for example, the minor jokes and digs that kids pass around to each other on social media. Sometimes they add up to something bigger because they are not just one-time events; they occur all day long, every day, because our children are spending countless hours on their devices. Gradually their brains and emotions absorb all of this content, making it seem real. Because the brains of kids are particularly impressionable, they no longer receive this continual stream of content as just "jokes." It is important that we expose our children to genuine, face-to-face interactions with us and their peers and keep them away from superficial interactions as best we can. This is critical if we want our children to develop strong, resilient minds.

Even the "happy" posts that our children's friends share about their vacations, sports performances, and social gatherings can have a negative impact. Because children are on the receiving end of hundreds, even thousands, of boastful photographs from their peers, it can cause them to start questioning the quality of their own life when compared to everyone else's. This overload on stimuli can lead to feelings of insecurity, because eventually the brain processes all of those self-indulgent photos and posts like this: *Everyone else's life is so much better than mine. I am such a loser! What is wrong with me?*

In a 2015 CNN documentary entitled *Being 13: Inside the Secret World of Teens*, one-third of the two hundred eighth graders who were polled spent a large portion of their social media time studying their friends' and peers' social media sites to figure out where they stood in the social pecking order. They looked to see who was in and who was out, whose popularity was growing and whose was slipping.[2]

A normal part of the adolescent stage of development is figuring out where one stands in the world, where one fits in. Spending hours and hours a day viewing everyone else's great life on Instagram and Snapchat can complicate this natural stage of development. Eventually our children will want to feel relevant too, and they will jump on board and start taking attention-seeking selfies and self-glorifying photos as a way of saying, "Hey, everyone, look at me; I have a life too." Unfortunately this plan never works, because feeling good about one's self and feeling accepted do not come from outside sources; they come from within.

Many children experience feelings of exclusion when they spend too much time using social media. Take, for example, a child who comes across a post about an after-school pool party they weren't invited to. If that child has insecurity issues, this can feel like a real slap in the face. Cue an emotional reaction that doesn't fit the crime. I've had dozens, maybe hundreds of students over the last couple of years who have come to my office, crying uncontrollably, after they discovered that they had been excluded from a get-together or an event. Obviously this is not a healthy way of handling this, but there's an explanation behind these extreme reactions.

Furthermore, I've received many phone calls from parents venting to me about situations just like this, where their child was left out of something. It can be very hard for some parents to hear this, because parents share in their children's pain, and they considered this to be a form of bullying. Usually these situations are nothing more than innocent oversights, yet bullying is also a factor. From my experience, bullying has taken on a whole new life and a whole new meaning.

BULLYING

My favorite television show as a child was *The Brady Bunch*. My siblings and I watched every episode. One episode that always stood out to me was the one where a boy named Buddy Hinton bullied Cindy Brady. Every day on Cindy's walk home from school, Buddy would be waiting for her in a specific location along her path to taunt Cindy and make fun of her lisp. Cindy felt helpless because Buddy was bigger than she was. Cindy's older brother Peter decided he would protect his younger sister and began walking her home from school. That didn't stop Buddy. When Peter tried to defend his sister, Buddy punched Peter, giving him a black eye.

Peter and Cindy's parents thought that "reasoning" was the best way to handle the situation. They called Buddy's parents, but there was no "reasoning" with Buddy's parents, so then Mr. and Mrs. Brady decided to teach Peter how to box. The following day, Buddy was waiting again. Buddy immediately started making fun of Cindy. Peter first tried to reason with Buddy, but Buddy would have none of it. Instead, Buddy took a swing at Peter, and Peter dodged the punch. He then took a swing of his own, landing a punch squarely on Buddy's mouth, knocking his tooth loose. Buddy wound up with a lisp of his own.

I like this story because it is a classic example of the school-yard bully learning his lesson after the victim defends himself. But the schoolyard bully is a thing of the past and has been replaced by screen bullies. Screen bullies are cowards who spew their venom through their handheld devices from the safety of their bedrooms. The difference between these two types of bullies is that the schoolyard bully can often be avoided by taking a different path. Screen bullies are everywhere and can attack all day, every day, from anywhere, without immediate consequences.

In 2011 the state of New Jersey, where I live and work, enacted The New Jersey Anti-Bullying Bill of Rights, the most comprehensive legislation in the country to combat bullying in New Jersey public schools. Every public school was required to appoint an "anti-bullying specialist" who would be responsible for investigating all acts of bullying. I was appointed to this role by the administration at my high school, and I have since investigated hundreds of bullying cases. Only a handful of them fit under the category of schoolyard bullying. Few of the bullying incidents I've investigated resemble the Buddy Hinton story. Nearly all of them involve social media or text messaging.

The types of comments and remarks that I have seen are beyond disturbing. For example, "Why don't you go kill yourself?" is on the tame end of the spectrum. I'm talking about comments that are so menacing I have to wonder how someone could bring themselves to treat another person this way. The comments and posts are so explicit that most of these kids would never have the guts to say the words face-to-face. The modern-day weapon of mass destruction, the smartphone, has made it easy for screen bullies to attack.

As my school's specialist, I take it as part of my mission to help kids who face bullying build their confidence. We teach kids not to bully others, to ignore bullies, and to report any incident of bullying. The ultimate message is about "anti-bullying." This is where I think some of the anti-bullying legislation misses the mark. I get it; we want to teach our kids to never bully or harass anyone, but we don't really teach them what to do if they are on the receiving end of bullying. "Just ignore the bully," or "Report it to an adult," we tell them. This is reactive and not very proactive. Personally I don't believe in "anti-anything"; I believe in "pro-everything." In other words, I believe in being proactive, being pro-confident, and teaching our children how to stand up for themselves. Bullies always have a big bark but a small bite. When they are confronted, nine times out of ten they back down. If we can teach children how to be confident, then they can't be bullied. Think about that for a minute. If a person is truly confident, is there really anything that anyone can say to them that is going to harm them? No. A confident kid recognizes that the bully's comments have nothing to do with them and everything to do with the bully's own insecurities.

Regardless, bullying is a real problem, and social media has a lot to do with it. Children who are more vulnerable, are trying to fit in, or crave attention are the perfect targets for screen bullies. They find themselves in online situations with other groups of kids and are not ready to handle the comments and remarks that may come.

How can we prevent our children from being bullied? First and foremost, we need to keep our kids away from social media. It is a breeding ground for screen bullies, and younger children in particular are not mature enough to handle the environment. Next, we need to continue to teach our children that the most important virtue is to love your neighbor as yourself and to treat everyone with kindness and respect. Finally, we need to teach kids on the receiving end of a bully's cowardly attacks that the bullying behavior has nothing to do with them and everything to do with the bully. Bullies are always insecure and lost. If we can teach our kids to understand this, they can learn to insulate themselves from the negative comments or actions of others.

When I was a kid, the biggest worry my friends and I had was getting picked last at Saturday pickup basketball games. We didn't have handheld battlefields where cowards could fire off their vitriolic comments. Instead we went to school, played outside, and just enjoyed being kids. There was no front-row ticket to everyone else's "better-than-yours" vacation at the beach or phenomenal performance at Saturday's soccer game. And parents had no outlet for showcasing their "special" child's straight As and wonderful life experiences. Life was simpler. The day-to-day, moment-to-moment details of our peers' lives were out of sight and therefore out of mind. Sure we got a little jealous if a kid from class homered in the championship game, but the envy was short-lived, it was normal, and it was part of being a kid. If anything, a little competition helped us learn, grow, and work harder. My experiences as a child didn't have a social media half-life the way children's experiences do today. A social media post that makes a child jealous or hurts their feelings can always be revisited, over and over again, leaving a lasting imprint on their mind.

Adolescent life is a lot different now. All of this exposure to everyone else's "perfect" life can cause confusion for kids, making them feel insecure about their own lives rather than grateful for them. The media, schools, and parents can further complicate this by pushing fairness and a victimization mentality rather than encouraging self-confidence and grit. We have created a trophy generation. Instead of insulating our kids from the superficial world of social media, we create rules to protect their self-esteem in that online environment, and it isn't working.

SELF-ESTEEM

Several years ago I coached my son's little league baseball team and often drove another kid, whom I'll call James, to practice. James, who was a fifth grader at the time, already owned a smartphone and would constantly use it in the back seat of my car whenever I drove him to practice. One day I asked him what he was doing on his phone all the time, and he responded, "I'm posting pictures on my Instagram account." When I asked him why he was doing that, he responded, "I don't know." But I knew. James wasn't an aspiring photographer attempting to share his artistic ability with others; James was seeking approval from others. He wanted to be noticed. He wanted to feel important. His young, vulnerable self-esteem was being flattered by artificial "likes," and he was setting himself up for some insecurity issues later on. Let me explain why.

The word *self* is the crucial part of the term self-esteem. We don't say *others*-esteem. But that is what is happening with our children. They often think that feeling good about themselves has something to do with how others perceive them. So instead of getting to know their true self—the person that they are—they compete with other kids to see who has the most likes. They actually believe that the number of likes they have is a reflection of who they are and a measure of their self-worth.

A study in the *Journal of Experiential Psychology* found that having a sense of purpose limits how reactive a person is to positive feedback on social media. Researchers defined a sense of purpose as ongoing motivation that is self-directed, oriented toward the future, and beneficial to others. Two groups were determined and examined, those with a high sense of purpose and those lacking a sense of purpose. All participants were asked to post a recent photo on social media and rate how they felt after getting a lot of likes or only a few likes. The participants with a high sense of purpose were unaffected by the amount of likes. The participants who did not have a high sense of purpose reported feeling a greater sense of self-esteem after receiving a lot of likes and a poorer sense of self-esteem when receiving few likes. Ultimately the study found that having a high sense of purpose keeps us emotionally steady, which is important for both academic and career success.[3]

Earlier in the book I mentioned my experience presenting to the freshman health classes at my school and how I believe their fatigue, lack of focus, and lethargy were because they were one of the first groups to get their first phone at an earlier age. In 2009, when I started lecturing about screens and electronics, my target audience was the parents of high school kids because that is where the problems existed at the time. Now the age that children are getting their first smartphones and using social media is getting younger and younger every year. How are younger and more vulnerable self-esteems going to hold up in that world of likes?

By 2014 my target audience had become mostly parents of eighth graders, because at the time that was around the age most kids were getting their first phones. Over the next several years my target audience became the parents of middle school children, sixth through eighth grade. Just recently, in March 2019, I gave my first lecture exclusively to parents of elementary-age children, kindergarten through fifth grade. When I arrived at the school that evening I was greeted by the principal and school counselor. After we struck up a conversation I was shocked to hear that many of the children in their school already had smartphones. I'm talking second and third graders. Let's be honest with ourselves: that's too young.

But what happens when everyone else's—I mean *everyone* else's—kids have phones? Well, all I can give you in that case is solidarity. And a commendation for standing your ground. When my son was in seventh grade, one of his friends invited him to a Super Bowl party. He had a great group of buddies who got together frequently. When I picked him up after the party, he didn't have the sparkle in his eyes that he normally had after spending time with friends. When I asked him how the party was, he said, "It was ok." As I pried a little deeper he told me that he didn't have that much fun because the six boys he was with were all using their smartphones the entire time the game was on. He was looking forward to watching the game and cheering with his friends, but he couldn't because he was the only one paying attention to the game. He felt alone. And he's not the only one. My daughter is currently in sixth grade and is one of only a few in her class not allowed to have a smartphone. Sometimes

I wonder if I should just get her a smartphone because she might become insecure as the "only kid" without one. But I refuse to give in. I refuse to raise my daughter to follow the crowd. So far she is more than fine; her self-esteem is firmly intact. Sure, she asks me to buy her a phone almost every day, and even says she will use her own money, but I simply use what I consider to be the most important word in the parental vocabulary—the word *no*.

FOMO

If this is the first time you're hearing the term FOMO, it is an acronym for Fear Of Missing Out. FOMO is a serious issue for preteens and teens because, as they become more enveloped in their digital interactions, the fear of missing something can cause legitimate anxiety. They become afraid to step away from a texting group chat, which can go on forever, because they fear they will become isolated or irrelevant. They crave the constant communication and attention, but the problem is that it isn't face-to-face, which is the only form of human interaction that can foster confidence, emotional regulation, and empathy. (I will explain this in more depth in chapter 7.) Furthermore, the text chats and social media posts can often become argumentative and downright abusive, which further damages kids' self-esteem.

Those kids who are immersed in the social-media world often stay up until the wee hours of the morning because they can't let go of the craving to be part of something. This causes sleep deprivation, academic issues, and subsequently anxiety and depression. A 2017 study that appeared in *Sleep Medicine* journal found that more adolescents in 2015 slept less than seven hours a night on most nights, and that smart-phones may be the cause.[4] The study sought to determine whether the self-reported sleep duration of US adolescents had changed as a result of new media screen time, and found that adolescents in 2015 compared to 2009 were around 17 percent more likely to report sleeping less than seven hours a night most nights. This was the time that handheld devices and social media began to increase significantly. Although this increase is concerning, I believe it is even worse than what the study found. Over the last few years I have asked hundreds of teenagers what time they go to bed at night. I have good relationships with these kids, and they know that what they tell me is anonymous. Most of them say that they go to bed somewhere between 1:00 a.m. and 3:00 a.m. every school night, and that their parents have no idea because once their parents fall asleep they go back on their devices or gaming consoles. Keep in mind that these students have to wake up by 6:00 or 6:30 in order to arrive to school by 7:30 when the homeroom bell rings.

WARNING SIGNS

Here are some warning signs that your child is spending too much time using any form of electronic media, including television, video games, handheld devices, and computers/tablets.

- Loses track of time when using electronic devices.
- Becomes agitated when interrupted.
- Prefers to spend time using electronics rather than being with friends or family in person.
- Does not follow time limits.

- Forms relationships with people online.
- Loss of interest in other activities.
- Seems restless when not using a device and preoccupied with getting back on.
- Avoids homework and chores because of spending too much time with electronics.
- Sneaks onto a device when no one is around and lies about it.

If your child exhibits any of these signs, you will need to step in. The best way to address any of these issues is to sit down with your child and express your concerns. Next, set strict guidelines for your child to follow and make it clear that if he or she violates them there will be consequences. Guidelines might include no electronics in the bedroom, no video games during the week, no smartphones in the car or during dinner, and mandatory unplugging times. Don't be convinced by the argument, "But my phone is my alarm!" Save their sleep—get them a real alarm clock instead of letting them use a device. Should your child violate any of the guidelines, you must hold them accountable and follow the consequences you prescribed. Consequences might include removing the television from the bedroom, taking away the cell phone for a week, or unplugging the video game console for a period of time. Consistency is the key.

CONSEQUENCES

Stephen was a seventeen-year-old high school junior when I started seeing him for counseling. Although his parents were married, they didn't see eye to eye and had very inconsistent parenting styles, which led to a lot of problems for Stephen. They were referred to me because Stephen continually got into trouble with his peers due to the inappropriate comments he posted on social media. Because Stephen's self-esteem was low he struggled to form friendships, and social media became his outlet. It was the perfect platform for him to express whatever he wanted to, which was often attention-seeking messages and photos, for which he received a tremendous amount of negative feedback from peers. But attention is attention. For some teenagers it doesn't matter if the attention is positive or negative; they are still being noticed, making them feel relevant instead of invisible.

After attending one of my lectures, Stephen's parents finally came to the realization that all of the time Stephen was spending on his computer and phone was significantly affecting him. He lied to them all the time about what he was doing in his online world. He would sneak the devices and use them when he was not permitted to. Even in the waiting room of my office, Stephen always wore a big pair of headphones and was totally disengaged from his parents, who were sitting right next to him. All of the deception that came from his social media addiction was having an enormous impact on his relationship with his parents.

After his parents informed me that they found inappropriate content on Stephen's phone directed toward a younger girl, I urged them to take away his devices. I explained to them that doing so would make things a lot worse at first, because he would undoubtedly become agitated, make threats, and try to manipulate them, which is exactly what he did. The day after our appointment Stephen's father called to tell me that Stephen had gone ballistic after they took away his devices. Words came out of his mouth that no parent could ever imagine, and he refused to go to school if his devices were not returned to him. He even threatened to harm himself. After a few days his parents couldn't take it any longer and gave him his devices back.

At our next session I urged Stephen to be very careful with any content he transmitted. Since he had just turned eighteen a couple of days before, I explained to him that he could get into a lot of trouble, particularly if he distributed any inappropriate content to a minor, because he was now a legal adult. He denied doing anything of the sort. Five days later, I learned from Stephen's parents that the police had arrived at their house with a search warrant to confiscate Stephen's laptop. A young girl had reported him to the police for making sexually explicit comments and more. Stephen was arrested and placed in jail. It was Stephen's poor self-esteem that led to these terrible consequences. In his online world he was relevant; people knew who he was, but that worked against him. Although Stephen's story is an extreme example of social media use gone bad, examples like this are very real. One bad decision can affect you for the rest of your life.

Although stories like Stephen's are just plain awful, it can be worse. Frightening new data about a dramatic rise in suicide rates among adolescents was recently published by the Centers for Disease Control and Prevention. In 1999 the death rate from traffic accidents for children ages ten to fourteen was quadruple the rate for suicide. Over the last fifteen years, the suicide rate for children in this age group has caught up to their death rate from traffic accidents. While the death rate from traffic accidents has been cut in half since 1999, the suicide rate has nearly doubled since 2007, leading to the crossover point. The CDC points to evidence that young adolescents are suffering from a range of health problems because of the country's rapidly changing culture. The pervasiveness of social media allows the entire school to witness someone's shame. And as children continue to have more access to new and different social media networks, the pressures continue when the child comes home from school. Although far more boys kill themselves than girls do, the CDC's data found that the suicide rate for girls has tripled while the rise for boys has increased by a third.[5] According to Rachel Simmons, the author of *Odd Girl Out: The Hidden Culture of Aggression in Girls*, "Social media is girl town."[6] Because girls statistically dominate visual platforms like Instagram and Facebook, Simmons states, they receive instant validation from peers and take things that were once private and make them public. For girls who are vulnerable, quantifying one's popularity through social media can be very destabilizing.

It seems that social media is even causing some crazy people to go to ultra-extreme measures to get a taste of "fame" and be noticed. I'm talking about desperate gunmen live-streaming their mass murders. One such story is that of Ian David Long. Long entered a country music bar in Southern California, opened fire, and killed twelve people. While in the bar he stopped shooting and posted to Instagram. Certainly this former Marine suffered from serious mental problems, but I'm sure social media didn't help. This is just one of many examples like this. Scary!

Folks, we have got to get a handle on this issue. We have to remember that we, the parents, are the ones who call the shots. If your child is the "only one" without a smartphone and all of the social media outlets it provides constant access to, good. Your child will be just fine. In fact they will be better than fine: they will develop a solid sense of self. If your child is obsessed with their smartphone and social media interactions, it is not too late to intervene. It won't be easy, but it is doable.

CHAPTER TIPS

1. Keep your children away from social media until late adolescence. They are not psychologically or emotionally ready to handle it.

2. If your child already has a device or social media access, make it clear to them that you will be checking it regularly. This is the greatest deterrent.

3. Constantly remind your children that a healthy self-esteem comes from their inside world, not their outside world. No amount of likes, follows, or streaks can fill up their self-esteem.

4. Have lots and lots of deep conversations with your children. There is no better way to help foster a strong self-esteem.

5. Do not allow your teenager to use their smartphone as an alarm clock. This is just an excuse for them to go on the device in their bedroom when you are sleeping. Get your teen a real alarm clock.

CHAPTER 4

The Multitasking Brains
of Kids

After just about every one of my parenting lectures, someone poses the following question: "Why does my child get four or five hours of homework a night?" My answer? *They don't!*

Your child probably has an hour or two of homework to do every night. They take so much longer to complete their work because they are multitasking while doing homework. That's right—kids are posting, texting, listening to music, watching YouTube, and doing homework simultaneously, and for some strange reason we ignore this. There's a lot of science that proves multitasking is no good; not only does it affect kids' schoolwork but it also affects their brains and bodies.

MEDIA MULTITASKING

A recent study consisting of twenty-two peer-reviewed research papers found that heavy media multitaskers performed worse on attention and working memory tests and in some cases had developed structural changes in the brain.[1] The study reviewed attention tests given to heavy multitaskers compared to light multitaskers. Heavy multitaskers are individuals who chronically switch back and forth from one type of electronic media to another much like the students I mentioned in the previous paragraph. Light multitaskers typically use just one form of electronic media, exclusively, without switching back and forth. The heavy multitaskers performed nearly 10 percent worse on the attention tests, and their ability to sustain attention was much poorer. The study also found that heavy multitaskers performed worse on working memory tests, which are linked to better focus and the ability to ignore distractions. Brain scans also showed that the anterior cingulate cortex, the area of the brain responsible for controlling attention, was smaller in heavy multitaskers.

The late Clifford Nass, a professor at Stanford University, conducted some of the most impressive research on multitasking. Nass defined multitasking as the use of unrelated media content. In other words, if a teenager listens to music while switching back and forth between Snapchat, text messages, and Instagram, they are multitasking between different, unrelated media content. Chronic task switching affects the front area of the brain that is responsible for executive functioning. This is the area of the brain that helps us organize our working memory, switch from one task to another smoothly, and focus on relevant information.[2]

Nass conducted experiments with his students that demonstrated how the frontal area of the brain is affected by multitasking. One of his experiments was simple. His students were asked to look at slides that consisted of two red rectangles and some blue rectangles; they were instructed to focus only on the red rectangles and determine how many times they rotated with each ensuing slide. Two groups of students participated: self-identifying high multitaskers and low multitaskers. The high multitaskers all believed that multitasking helped them perform better academically, but the experiment proved them wrong. High multitaskers struggled immensely with this simple experiment when more blue rectangles were added from slide to slide. Their brains could not help but get distracted by the blue rectangles, and the more that were added the worse they did. Low multitaskers were unaffected by the blue rectangles, no matter how many were added. They were able to focus on the red rectangles as instructed and accurately determine how many times the red rectangles rotated.

Nass decided to further prove his theory with another experiment that included the use of an fMRI (functional magnetic resonance imaging) device. In the experiment both groups were given a simple task-switching exercise while connected to the fMRI device, and the results were impressive. High multitaskers used twenty times more of their brain while engaging in the experiment than low multitaskers. But there was an unforeseen outcome: they were using the wrong part of the brain, the part known as the visual cortex. Low multitaskers needed only a small amount of brainpower to complete the task, and it was the area of the brain they were supposed to be using, the prefrontal cortex. In other words, the high multitasking students were actually worse at task multitasking than the low multitasking students.

Imagine how hard it must be for high multitasking students to listen in class or focus on completing homework efficiently and effectively when their brains don't work that way. They struggle immensely. I can tell you that it isn't teachers giving too much homework that is causing so many kids to "have too much homework."

Here is an example. Nass used another experiment, a classic one created by Daniel J. Simons, called "the monkey business illusion." Before you continue to read, navigate to this link and follow the instructions in the video: http://bit.ly/M9rlws.

How did you do? Did you guess the correct number of passes? If not, you are probably a high multitasker. If you succeeded, then you are likely a low multitasker.

In case you did not get a chance to try the experiment, here's how it works: As the video begins there are six young ladies standing in a line. Three are wearing white shirts and one is holding a basketball. The other three are wearing black shirts and one is holding a basketball. In the experiment you are asked to count how many times the players in white pass the basketball back and forth to each other. What makes the task challenging is that the girls wearing black are also passing the ball among each other, which can be distracting. As all six are passing the ball to their respective teammates, they are also walking between one another, making it even more confusing. High multitaskers fail miserably at counting the correct number of passes between the girls wearing white because their brains can't help but be distracted by the players in black, along with other distractions happening in the video. Low multitaskers have no problem counting the correct number of passes.

Nass's experiment emphasized another difference between high and low multitaskers' brains. In the video, while the basketball is passed around between players on both teams, there are three other things occurring. First, a person wearing a black gorilla suit walks right through the group of young ladies. Next, one of the girls wearing black leaves the stage. Lastly, the curtain in the background changes color. Watch the video again and see for yourself. High multitaskers were good at noticing the gorilla and the other anomalies but were bad at correctly counting the number of passes between the players wearing white. Low multitaskers were good at counting the passes correctly but did not notice the gorilla, the girl in black leaving the stage, or the curtain changing colors.

Ultimately, high multitaskers were bad at managing memory. If you look at the brain as a file cabinet that neatly stores necessary information, the brains of high multitaskers are a mess. The executive functioning area of the brain is compromised.

Researchers have also conducted studies with drivers. They looked at MRIs of drivers to see how much brain attention went toward driving. When another bit of information was layered in, like music on the radio, the amount of brain bandwidth going toward driving dropped by 37 percent.[3] So the drivers aren't really multitasking but rather are paying less attention to driving. Have you ever tried watching a movie while simultaneously scanning through Facebook? It's almost impossible to pay attention to the movie.

A guidance counselor where I work invited me to a meeting recently with a concerned mom. The mom was worried about her fourteen-year-old daughter's academic struggles. The girl's teachers also attended the meeting. The mom explained that although her daughter was a smart girl, she often became overwhelmed and would shut down. The mom also explained that a simple fifteen-minute homework assignment took her daughter two hours to complete, and the girl agreed that her mother wasn't exaggerating.

The girl's math teacher spoke first, stating that the girl was always distracted by her laptop. The teacher constantly had to tell her to close it. (In my school district, each student is provided with a personal laptop.) Every teacher who spoke agreed that the laptop was a major distraction for the girl. After the teachers gave their accounts, I chimed in and asked the mom if her daughter was distracted by her smartphone or laptop while doing homework. The mom stated that she was.

This brief meeting told me a lot. Here I had a fourteen-year-old girl whose brain was all over the place. She had over twenty missing homework assignments because she forgot about them, and it took her hours to complete simple assignments that should have taken minutes. Her brain's file cabinet, her prefrontal cortex, was a disorganized mess. Her constant switching between computer, phone, and social media was dividing her attention across many different types of stimuli, reducing her ability to focus on one specific task: schoolwork. Rather than processing material and storing it in her long-term memory bank, this girl was sending the information from all of these different sources, including schoolwork, to the wrong part of her brain. The scattered information could not be stored long-term and retrieved later.

If you talk to any veteran high school or college English teacher, they'll tell you that many of their current students struggle to produce essays that are well organized and logically argued. Essays are often patchy and disorganized because they are composed by students who have their phones nearby constantly lighting up with notifications and alerts.

This continual switching between writing and checking the phone interrupts the process of writing and leads to papers that miss the fundamental essentials of proper writing: an introductory statement, a body, and a conclusion.

POOR FOCUS

Multitasking can also cause fragmented thinking. Because tweets, posts, texts, and likes are all performed in short, quick bursts, over time the brain becomes accustomed to this type of communication. The brain learns to think in a fragmented way. Dr. Gary Small says, "It's a basic principle that the brain is very sensitive to any kind of stimulation, and from moment to moment, there is a very complex cascade of neurochemical electrical consequences to every form of stimulation. If you have repeated stimuli, your neural circuits will be excited. But if you neglect other stimuli, other neural circuits will be weakened."[4]

A research study conducted by the University of London shows just how damaging multitasking can be. The study revealed that participants who multitasked during cognitive tasks experienced IQ score declines that were similar to what researchers would expect to see if the study subjects had smoked marijuana or stayed up all night. IQ drops of 15 points for multitasking adults lowered their scores to the average range of an eight-year-old child. Bestselling author of *Emotional Intelligence 2.0*, Dr. Travis Bradberry, comments, "The next time you're writing your boss an email during a meeting, remember that your cognitive capacity is being diminished to the point that you might as well let an eight-year-old write it for you."[5]

Washington Post writer Jeff Guo contends that students should never use laptops to take notes. According to Guo's article, economists from West Point conducted a large experiment to demonstrate how classroom computing affects learning. They randomly banned computers from some sections of a popular economics course at the military academy. One-third of the cadets were allowed to use laptops or tablets for note-taking during lectures, one-third could use them only to look at class material, and one-third were prohibited from using any technology. Not surprisingly, the students who were allowed to use laptops or tablets did worse on the final exam. Interestingly, the smartest students seemed to be harmed the most. Among the students with the highest ACT scores, those who were allowed to use laptops or tablets performed significantly worse than their peers in the no-technology section. What's odd about these results is that one would expect the smartest students who were in the laptop-friendly section to use these machines more prudently. Instead, they were the biggest victims of technology because they overestimated their ability to multitask. Or, as Guo states, "The top students might have had the most to gain by paying attention in class."[6]

Another way to interpret the West Point results is by using the cadets' average score on the math section of the SAT, which was 511 out of 800. According to Guo, "The difference between exam grades in the laptop-friendly sections and exam grades in the no-laptop sections is the equivalent to the difference between scoring a 511 and scoring a 491 on the SAT's math section. (That's roughly the same boost a high school student might expect from hiring an SAT tutor.)"[7] This is more evidence that multitasking doesn't work. Guo then warns,

"Beware of people who take laptops into meetings—even to take notes, because they're probably not listening to you."[8] Multitasking is bad not only for kids but for adults too.

A study published in *Psychological Science* supports the West Point findings. This study sought to test how note-taking by hand or by computer affected learning. The researchers selected university students and asked them to take notes from a series of TED talks they were shown. The students who used a laptop to take notes did substantially poorer in answering conceptual-application questions about the talks when compared to students who took notes by hand. The evidence suggested that taking notes by hand produced superior external storage as well as superior encoding functions when compared to taking notes with a laptop.[9] In other words, our brains are much better at learning and retaining information when we take notes by hand as opposed to using a computer.

OTHER EFFECTS

Common Sense Media's 2014 white paper—which reviews existing studies on media use, technology, and addiction—concludes that there is cause for concern with regard to the overuse of screen media because of the potentially damaging consequences. The paper found that multitasking, which is common for kids doing homework and socializing, affects learning, schoolwork, and memory. Too much media use can also undermine empathy and reduce face-to-face conversation.

What else does screen time do to kids' brains? A landmark study by the National Institute of Health, which began in 2018, is attempting to see how tablets, smartphones, and other screens are impacting adolescent brain development. Over the next decade, $300 million will be spent to follow eleven thousand kids through their adolescent years. Scientists began by interviewing nine- and ten-year-olds and scanning their brains. On *60 Minutes*, Anderson Cooper sat down with some of the researchers to get a glimpse at what they've learned so far.[10] The first to be interviewed was Dr. Gaya Dowling, who brought the first wave of data from the brain scans of 4,500 participants to the table. The MRIs showed a premature thinning of the cortex in some kids who spent more than seven hours a day on screens. The cortex is the outermost layer of the brain that processes information from the five senses. Some of the preliminary data in the study has also revealed that kids who spend more than two hours a day on screens received lower scores on thinking and language tests.

According to Dr. Dimitri Christakis, another researcher, "In many ways, the concern that investigators like me have is that we're sort of in the midst of a natural kind of uncontrolled experiment on the next generation."[11] Dr. Christakis is one of the few scientists to have already done experiments on how screens impact the brain development of children under age two. He's also the lead author of the American Association of Pediatrics' most recent guidelines for screen time, which now recommends no screen time at all, except for video chatting, for children under twenty-four months. Dr. Christakis believes that children under two are much more vulnerable to become addicted to smartphones or tablets than teenagers because the experience is much more gratifying for children that young. Electronic devices are simply more engaging than any traditional toy—and according to Tristan Harris, a former Google manager, they are purposely designed that way.

Harris explained to Cooper that there is a whole playbook of techniques tech developers use to get people, including children, to use their products for as long as possible. Harris was one of the first Silicon Valley insiders to publicly acknowledge that phones and apps are being designed to grasp as much of our children's attention as possible. He calls it a war for attention and worries that it may be affecting children. When Cooper asked Harris if parents understood the complexities of this, Harris stated, "No. And I think this is really important. Because there's a narrative that, oh, I guess they're just doing this like we used to gossip on the phone, but what this misses is that your telephone in the 1970s didn't have a thousand engineers on the other side of the telephone who were redesigning it to work with other telephones and then updating the way your telephone worked every day to be more and more persuasive."[12]

Finally, Anderson Cooper interviewed Roxy Shimp, an eighteen-year-old who agreed to have her brain scanned as she followed Instagram. As expected, the feel-good part of Shimp's brain, the part that releases dopamine, lit up during the experiment. Dopamine is a brain chemical that plays a pivotal role in cravings and desire. Tech developers want to activate this chemical as much as possible to create a craving and secure our addiction to their products.

· · · · ·

Multitasking and too much screen time in general affects children's attention, grades, test scores, and brains, but there's one last area I'd like to touch on—their waistlines. According to an April 2019 article in *Brain Imaging and Behavior*, chronic switching from gadget to gadget can impair self-control when it comes to eating, making it harder to resist the temptation to snack on unhealthy foods.[13] According to the lead author, Richard Lopez, "Increased exposure to phones, tablets and other portable devices has been one of the most significant changes to our environments in the past few decades, and this occurred during a period in which obesity rates also climbed in many places."[14] In this study, 123 young adults ages eighteen to twenty-three were surveyed to assess their levels of media multitasking and distractibility. Those individuals who showed higher levels of multitasking had higher body mass indexes (BMI) and higher body fat, and they tended to spend more time at campus cafeterias than non-multitaskers. Brain scans showed that the part of the brain associated with food temptation showed a higher level of activity when high multitaskers saw images of food.

There is nothing good about multitasking—that constant switching between media that takes up so much of our children's precious time. It affects just about every aspect of our children's well-being, from their brains to their emotions to their physical bodies. Fortunately, there are some strategies you can implement to prevent this. Here are some tips to start with.

CHAPTER TIPS

1. Have a conversation with your children about everything you learned in this chapter. Encourage them to read the information carefully.
2. Never allow your children to have a smartphone anywhere near them while doing homework.

3. If your child uses a laptop to do homework, make sure all alerts are turned off.

4. Do not allow your children to listen to music while doing homework. Parents ask me all the time if this is ok, as many kids have become accustomed to doing this. I would discourage this practice.

5. When your children are watching television, prohibit other electronic devices from being used simultaneously.

6. Practice what you preach.

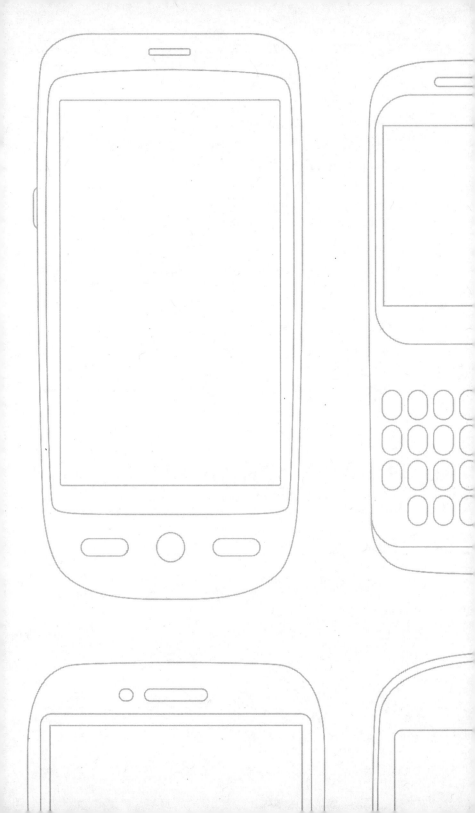

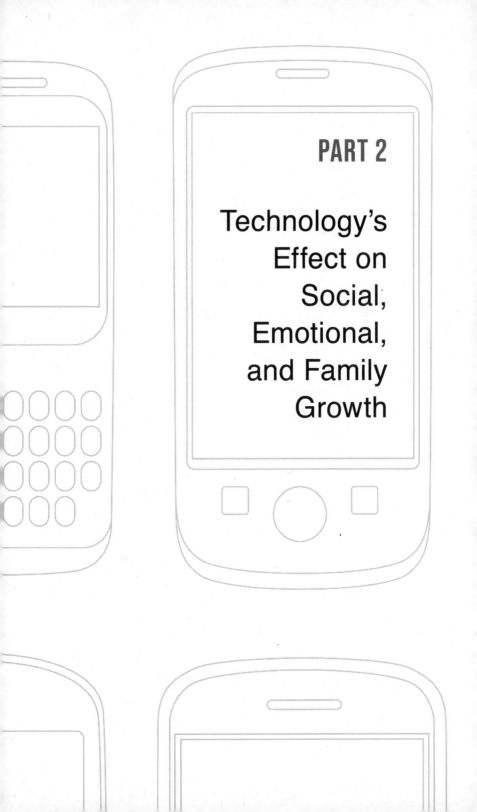

PART 2

Technology's Effect on Social, Emotional, and Family Growth

CHAPTER 5

Gamer Kids

The Great Human Disconnect

Alex was a sixteen-year-old high school junior who hadn't been to school in six weeks. After the school psychologist, assistant principal, and I met with his father it became obvious what the problem was: video games. Alex spent so much time playing video games that he'd become a full-blown addict. According to his father, Alex played for a minimum of twelve hours per day, seven days a week. Alex gained a lot of weight and became depressed, which contributed to his anxiety and subsequent school avoidance. The video games that were once just a pastime had become a drug for him. Everything around him began to crumble—school, health, family, and social life. Interestingly, his father didn't connect the dots until after our meeting; he did not realize that Alex's video game obsession was the source of his problems.

You may be wondering how a parent could allow a child to play twelve hours of video games each day. You'd be surprised how many parents are oblivious to the amount of time their children spend gaming. Alex's father presumed that because his son was home all the time he was simply bored and had nothing else to do to pass the time. He didn't understand that it was the other way around. Being home with all of that free time didn't lead to Alex's video game addiction; his video game addiction trapped him at home and disconnected him from the world outside of his bedroom.

A couple of years ago I received a phone call from the parents of a seventeen-year-old boy who was referred to me by someone who attended one of my lectures. They wanted to schedule an appointment to discuss options for their video game–addicted son. The session I had with them was troubling. Their son had not been to school in over two years and was receiving home instruction. He barely ate and had lost a tremendous amount of weight because he was unable to pull himself away from his gaming console.

The boy's video gaming had gotten so out of control when he was in middle school that by the time he reached high school, he refused to attend. Any time his parents attempted to take away his beloved video game console he would react dramatically. He punched holes in walls and became verbally and physically violent. His parents were scared of their son and called the police on several occasions. The saddest part was that the couple had separated and was pursuing divorce because addressing their son's addiction had put so much stress on their marriage. At the time of our visit, their son was a full-blown agoraphobic; he hadn't left the house in months. I never got a chance to help the boy because his parents were unable to get him to my office.

NO EASY SOLUTIONS

When parents call me for help with their video game–addicted children, I know they are hoping I have some magic powers that will make the problem go away. What I've learned from my experiences is that most parents of video game addicts are afraid to take away the games for fear of what the child might do. The child's reaction often resembles that of a crack addict whose drugs have been taken away. One parent told me that after her son started failing all of his classes she decided it was time to unplug the Xbox. Her son—whom she and his teachers described as calm, friendly, and respectful—went nuts. He cursed her out, destroyed the coffee table in the family room, and punched holes in his bedroom wall. Another mother told me that after she removed her son's games, he took a knife out of the kitchen drawer and threatened to stab her with it. And still other parents have told me that when they've taken away their child's games, their child threatened to commit suicide. There is something gravely wrong here. And many of you reading this know exactly what I am talking about because you have experienced similar situations with your own sons and daughters.

The addicted teen-gamer is not only a national problem; it's an international one. Taiwan, for example, has an epidemic of gaming addicts, which has prompted the government to create laws that hold parents accountable if their children spend too much time gaming.[1] Some other Asian countries have created military-style boot camp rehabilitation centers for video game–addicted kids. There are stories of teenagers soiling themselves and nearly starving themselves because they were unable to detach themselves from their games, even for just a few minutes. One Asian teen was so addicted to his video games that he chopped off his own hand so that he could stop playing. Thankfully, doctors were able to reattach it.[2]

Video game addiction causes reclusiveness and social anxiety, and many gaming addicts socialize with "friends" through headsets and have no real-life social interactions. Parents across the world feel paralyzed, fearing that if they take away the games then their children will become lonely and depressed because they will have no one to associate with and nothing to do.

Many of the preteens and teens I counsel are well aware of their gaming addiction and the impact it is having on their lives, yet they still can't get themselves to stop playing. As parents, we must step in and take control of these situations no matter how difficult they are.

Here are some comments from real teenagers:

> I am 14 and I'm a freaking addict . . . my parents seem to care but never try to kick me off or even try to help. I have 2 lvl 70s one that is full t6 and other full t5. Thus I have no life. I can't even imagine what I would do if I deleted my toons. I really want to quit but I can't. I mean this [expletive deleted] game is controlling me and I can't stop. I have almost deleted my toons but I'm afraid I'll just start up another one.

> I'm 12 and I can't stop playing. Wow I play about 8–10 hours a day mostly because all my friends are on it, and I'm bored when I don't play. I just failed socials too so what should I do?

> WOW addiction is no joke. I started to play because cousins and friends played (who are by the way all overweight). At first all I did was play WOW (World of Warcraft) once or twice a

day for let's say 2–3 hours. Then out of the blue my cousin stopped playing because he said he was addicted to WOW, so he gave me his 70 (rogue). Well after that I was on 6–10 hours a day. I ignored my friends, went from working out 4 times a week to twice. I would cuss people who asked me to get off. In the end though I realized by playing WOW I was just supporting big business. Also, why waste money, time with friends for a game? I know people who would be a lot better off without WOW. I just want to try to get all the money I have invested into it back so I am going to sell the (rogue).

I want to quit WOW so badly. I've been playing for 2 years. . . . The problem is that I don't know what else to do besides play video games.

I ended up ill with a deep vein thrombosis in one of my legs caused, according to the doctors, by me sitting on my backside doing instances all night and all day.[3]

According to the NPD Group, a market research company, there are thirty-four million hardcore gamers who spend an average of twenty-two hours a week in front of the screen. China and the United States claim 50 percent of the world's gaming revenues, and by 2018 the video gaming market had reached $135 billion.[4] The *Diagnostic and Statistical Manual* (*DSM-V*), which is published by the American Psychological Association (APA) and offers common language and standard criteria for the classification and diagnosis of mental disorders, describes internet gaming disorder as a "condition for further study." In other words, it is on the APA's radar.

Can gaming really be considered an addiction? People ask me this question all the time, and I can finally say for certain that my answer is yes. In June 2018 the World Health Organization (WHO), in its latest revision to its disease classification manual, added "gaming disorder" as a separate addiction. CBS covered this story, and according to Dr. Shekhar Saxena, the director of the WHO's mental health and substance abuse department, "The agency accepted the proposal that gaming disorder should be listed as a new problem based on scientific evidence, citing 'the need and demand for treatment in many parts of the world.'"[5] Experts who were interviewed by CBS supported the WHO's decision and shared stories of students dropping out of school and entire family structures falling apart. Cam Adair, founder of the website *Game Quitters*, told CBS that gaming ultimately caused him to drop out of high school. He was pretending to have jobs while in reality he played video games up to sixteen hours a day. When he finally realized he had a problem, he wrote a suicide note. Thankfully, he has overcome his addiction and is on a mission to help others.

CBS news also caught up with Dr. Mark Griffiths. Griffiths, who has been researching video gaming disorder for thirty years, said, "Video gaming is like a non-financial kind of gambling from a psychological point of view. Gamblers use money as a way of keeping score whereas games use points."[6] Griffiths explained that gaming prompts a neurological response that influences feelings of pleasure and reward and can lead to addictive behavior. Being engrossed in games affects the same area of the brain as drug use.

The WHO's reason for classifying gaming disorder as a disease is plausible. As I've noted, I've worked with many families that have been torn apart because of gaming addiction. I've also received emails from people all over the world telling me their personal stories about how gaming has ruined their life or destroyed their family. I'd like to share with you the most extreme example of gaming addiction I've ever heard. This is an actual email I received from a woman who saw me on television talking about gaming addiction. She gave me permission to share her story but asked that I not use her name. Please keep in mind that this is an extreme outcome of a gaming addiction and is very unlikely to happen to even the most addicted gamers—but it is possible.

> I just watched your program on Tucker Carlson . . . long story short my daughter became addicted to Minecraft at age 13 and disassociated with the real world as we know it and brainwashed herself into believing Minecraft was the real world and in 2016 at age 15 she took her life by hanging herself at a playground in order to go to Minecraft world. I'm a very private person and I never talk about what perpetuated her death as it would sound too bizarre to be believable but I've been on a crusade for years to find answers. Regards—B

During our email exchange B also told me that before her daughter became obsessed with Minecraft, she was a great student and a loving child. After she started playing the game, she lost her sense of reality and thought that the fairy princess of Minecraft was her leader. B believes that too many kids are vulnerable to being brainwashed by these games when they are too innocent to really think for themselves, and I agree. This poor woman is forever heartbroken and is convinced that the images and messages from these games can trigger underlying mental health conditions. She wanted to share this information to help others so that her daughter's death is not in vain, and she fears that our youth are heading in a bad direction with the constant messages and images they see on screens—and that cases like hers will increase dramatically if parents continue to remain ignorant.

FORTNITE FIXATION

Are we ignorant? I think many parents are but don't realize it; they simply don't understand the depths of gaming addiction. I'd be remiss if I did not talk a little bit about Fortnite. If you have a son, chances are he plays Fortnite; your daughter might too. What's the craze about Fortnite? Fortnite has quickly become one of the most popular online games in history with close to 250 million downloads as of April 1, 2019. This shooter game uses savvy graphics that include cool dance moves, pop culture, and humor. The game's animations are broadly appealing to youth everywhere.

Although there isn't much blood and gore in Fortnite, the object of the game is to kill before being killed, to be the last one standing just like in *The Hunger Games*. Fortnite has a PEGI rating of 12, meaning it is meant for players ages twelve and older. However, I have come across many cases of players younger than twelve—even as young as six. I'm surprised by this, considering its violent nature and reports of online predators using the game's chat function to connect with children.

Although Fortnite is free, its creator, Epic Games, makes money through in-game purchases of attire and "emotes" and "skins." These add-ons don't increase the player's chances of winning, but they do make their avatar appear cool, something that is quite tempting for children. Skins are the avatar bodies that players use, while emotes are the various actions that the avatars can perform. These variables, combined with the fast-paced nature of the game, trigger the body's hormones, like adrenaline. The player gets a rush and their heart starts racing as they get into the game. With some practice, the game isn't all that hard to win, and when a player finally does win, there is a big payoff as dopamine, the brain's feel-good chemical, is released—and the player craves more; they want to keep activating the brain's natural reward system because it feels great. This is the same reward system that is tied to every addiction, including drugs. The game developers know exactly what they are doing.

Much like any addiction, when gaming begins to interfere with important life areas such as relationships, health, or school, we know it has become a serious problem. Gaming can pose self-esteem and relationship issues as well because it can allow players to act differently than they would normally act in real life. A shy kid can become unreserved, and a timid kid can become aggressive.

Many socially challenged kids I've counseled over the years discover the virtual world of gaming, where they can be more expressive and powerful, leading armies into victory. Playing these video games creates a feeling of real accomplishment even though there is nothing real about it. In fact, the same neurons in the brain that would fire after actually hitting a game-ending home run in real life can also fire through maneuvering a game controller. Many parents of gaming-addicted kids have told me that their child has no real friends because no one calls, no one comes over to the house, and no one invites their child anywhere. The thought of taking the games away is a tough one because some parents feel that by doing so they are taking away the only "friends" their child has and the only thing their child is good at.

Sadly, a child who spends all of their time socializing through a headset and screen and no time engaged in face-to-face interaction will not develop the necessary communication skills required to succeed in the real world. For kids like these just the thought of face-to-face interaction can cause serious distress. It goes back to the science of neuroplasticity—if you don't use certain skills, you lose them. Furthermore, if virtual success from being good at a specific video game is the only feeling of success your child has, you can bet that their self-esteem will continue to suffer.

PHYSICAL REALITIES

A study published in the journal *Plos One* found that sleep deprivation caused by video game addiction may increase obesity and lead to cardio-metabolic deficits. In the study, researchers collected data from ninety-four adolescents between the ages of twelve and seventeen. They used surveys, Fitbit sleep monitors, physical exams, and blood tests. After analyzing all of the data, the researchers concluded that video game addiction was negatively associated with sleep duration, which was related to an elevation in blood pressure, LDL cholesterol, triglycerides, and high insulin resistance. Ultimately, video game addiction can lead to obesity, heart disease, and type II diabetes.[7]

In light of all of these consequences, mental and physical, you may be wondering if your child suffers from gaming addiction. If you are concerned that your child may be a video game addict, look for these warning signs:

- Spends the majority of hours outside of school on the computer or other gaming system
- Has a drop in grades
- Lacks focus in school
- Sleeps in school
- Lies about video game playing
- Chooses to socialize with video game friends instead of real friends
- Lacks real friends
- Drops out of sports and extracurricular activities
- Throws tantrums when told to turn off games
- Becomes irritable when not playing games

If you are the parent of a child who spends too much time playing video games but are afraid that unplugging these games is going to make matters worse, it is a risk you are going to have to take. Yes, your child may throw a tantrum and make your life miserable, but this will not last forever. Later, you will be thankful that you chose to act. For many years I have been advising parents to pull the plug on video games. See what happens after thirty days, I tell them. Many parents have come back to me with stories about the remarkable changes they've seen from their child after doing this. One particular mom who attended one of my lectures tried it, and she has allowed me to share her story:

Matthew's Journey: A Story of Electronics Addiction and Recovery by Cynthia McNulty

My nine-year-old son, Matthew, is an addict. Matthew is addicted to video games and electronics. And although it might not sound like a big deal, it is. On Super Bowl Sunday, I allowed my son to binge play on his iPad so I could watch the game without being disturbed. He was out of my hair, quiet and happy, so why not? What happened after that is why I will never allow that to happen again.

My son has ADHD, which is difficult to manage on a regular day. Throw in an overdose of electronics and it is a recipe for disaster. After the Super Bowl ended and his gaming session was over, he could not get himself to sleep. This is something that had never been an issue before. He was so overstimulated that he was unable to regulate his body, behavior, and mood, which caused him to be nasty, irritable, and downright miserable. The next two days were an absolute nightmare, not only because I did not allow him to play video games during this time but also because he was coming down from the negative effects of binge playing. He was truly having symptoms of addiction withdrawal.

Rewind to the week prior. I took my son to see a presentation called "Digitally Distracted" by Thomas Kersting about the negative effects that electronics have on the brain. During the presentation, Mr. Kersting listed warning signs of your child having an addiction: loses track of time when on electronics, becomes agitated when interrupted, prefers to spend time using electronics rather than playing, does not follow time limits, loses interest in other activities, seems restless when not using a device and preoccupied with getting back on, avoids homework and chores because of spending too much time with electronics, and sneaks a device when no one is around and lies about it.

Throughout the entire presentation, Matthew sat with his arms crossed while glaring at me. He did not want to be there. So I was surprised when, during the car ride home, he stated, "I am addicted to video games." He was neither angry nor argumentative. He did not yell or say it in a mean tone. As a matter of fact, he was very quiet, as if reflecting on what the presenter had to say. I was completely taken aback that he recognized this within himself. Isn't admitting you have an addiction the first step to healing? I knew then that I had to take action. I was relieved that he understood what was going on and acknowledged his feelings, and told him that we would make a plan to help him.

I was like a lot of parents when it comes to video games. I didn't believe I was permissive or overindulgent with electronics. I set boundaries. I was that mom who only allowed video games on the weekends, and maybe, if he earned it, an hour a day after school. But, when I looked at things honestly, it was much more.

He would bring a device to school, which meant he was spending time on his electronics during morning care before school, at recess, and during after school care. When we were out to dinner, he was allowed to play on a device while we waited for the food. On the weekends, I would set a timer for an hour, but after him not abiding by it and then negotiating, one hour would turn into two hours easily, twice a day. At times I would stand my ground and fight with him to turn it off, but other days I just did not have the energy. Especially if I was cooking, doing laundry, or simply reading a book. Sometimes it was easier to just let it go because I had time to myself, and he was being quiet.

But after sitting through that presentation, and then seeing the very real-world consequences come to life with my son [after the Super Bowl], I knew we had to make some serious changes.

Even with all this information staring me in the face, I still contemplated allowing him some gaming time on the weekends because I dreaded his reaction and I did not want to have to deal with it. Plus, I was a little lost as to even where or how to start this detox plan. And then I realized, like with any addiction, I needed to seek help from a professional. Luckily, because of Matthew's ADHD, we already had a relationship with a cognitive behavior therapist. After I told her about Matthew's comment to me after the presentation and then relayed the events of Super Bowl Sunday, she gave me very sound advice. "If he was addicted to drugs or alcohol, would you still let him have just a little bit?" she asked. At that moment, I truly understood that this was a real addiction, just like any other, and decided to completely cut Matthew off from all of his electronics cold turkey. No iPad, no DS, no Xbox, no computer, no Nintendo Switch, no access to my phone. Nothing.

The first week was absolute torture. Initially, he thought he was going to be able to handle it, probably thinking I would eventually give in. But after twenty-four hours of no electronics, withdrawal set in. And it was a true addict's withdrawal. His morning and night routines were awful. He was so angry at me and so mean to me that I often cried on the way to work. He fought, cried, screamed, begged, and asked every ten minutes. At one point he got so angry that he trashed his room, something that he had only done once before, which had also been in reaction to the consequence of losing access to video games. I lost my cool and yelled at him. It would have been easy to give up here, and I came close to my breaking point, but I thought back to the question that the therapist asked me and found the strength to say no.

After about five days of anger, his emotions transitioned from anger to sadness. For about four days, when he asked for his electronics and was told no, he no longer stomped off angry but cried instead. And as he went through his emotional process, so did I. I questioned myself constantly and wondered if I was doing the right thing, day after day. Still, I kept thinking about the doctor's words, and how this would not only help Matthew now but also in the future.

In order to combat some of these emotions, we created a list of fun things to do instead. Slime, puzzles, board games, cards, coloring, mazes, word searches. You name it, we did it. I became his playmate. We played a new board game daily and became experts at playing cards. My involvement was completely hands-on. When it was time to cook, he helped peel potatoes. When I had to do laundry, he poured the detergent. He was kept busy all day. Every time he was "bored," I referred him to the list. Sometimes he entertained himself, but many times he searched for a social interaction with me, his father, or his sisters. This was probably even more exhausting than listening to him cry and complain because I needed to keep him occupied. These were the moments that I wanted to bend the rules and allow him to play for a little while because I just wanted some time to myself. Thankfully I held strong and did not give in. Because despite the anger and sadness that he experienced, and the frustration that I experienced, as we started to spend more one-on-one time together without the distraction of electronics, we began to also experience moments of joy. Laughter while playing a game. Or a sense of connection while he helped me with chores. And just the genuine closeness that you can't have unless you are fully present with the other person.

Around the third week, acceptance began to set in. He began to admit to people that he was in a video game detox. Family members started taking notice that he was more present and conversational. He was and is a happier, friendlier, funnier, more pleasant Matthew. He feels better about himself and admits he doesn't miss it. Occasionally he will ask to have access to his electronics, and when he is told no, he still sometimes gets angry, but when I remind him of how great he feels and that I am proud of him, he lets it go.

Matthew has not had access to video games or electronics for four weeks now. Not that we haven't had missteps. He played on an iPad at a friend's house for about thirty or forty-five minutes on day twenty-four of his detox, but that did not seem to set him back at the time. However, two days later he asked again, and we got into an argument over the reason why he could not have access. More tears, more frustration. He was very persistent and only wanted to play for fifteen minutes. I was on the verge of saying yes, because this entire experience has been hard for both of us, and I was tired, but I knew if I gave in fifteen minutes would turn into more. So I tried to keep my focus on the end goal, knowing that if I could stay strong, this would pass. I pulled out a deck of cards and started playing by myself, and soon enough he was right next to me having a good time.

Because of his addiction, electronics limitations have been placed on our entire family (my husband and myself, and Matthew's two older sisters). But rather than being resentful, we find that the bond this has created for us has enriched all our lives. When we go out for dinner, instead of looking at our phones we talk to each other and find things to laugh about. If there is a lull in the conversation, we play cards or Spot It while we wait for our food. Board games are an everyday occurrence in our house now. We are happier and more socially connected to each other, and we enjoy each other's company so much more. And we are all so proud of Matthew.

As necessary as this journey has been, by no means has it been easy, and I'm not sure that it ever will be. There were moments I wanted to give up and give in, and I continue to fight that battle, particularly when I'm tired and frustrated and just want some time to myself. I was angry with myself and my child for allowing this to happen. I was resentful of other parents who didn't have to go through this, and of their kids who seemingly dangled electronics in my son's face. I was frustrated at the school for allowing students to bring in their handheld video games. I hated that I cared so much. And I still fear that my son may have an addictive personality and worry what future challenges he may have.

Will I be able to keep electronics away from him forever? I realistically know that I cannot. What I hope Matthew does learn from this, though, is that he can live a fun, happy life without electronics being a priority or a crutch. Like any addiction, recurrence is very real when surrounded by your vice. I hope that, eventually, Matthew can develop a healthy relationship with his electronics without addiction setting back in. And while I'm realistic that this will be a process full of pitfalls, I'm hopeful that we can figure out a way forward, knowing how far we've come.

Electronics addiction is very real, particularly for children and their developing brain. And it can have lifelong repercussions if it is not addressed. I hope I wasn't too late helping my son. I hope that we both have the strength to continue to fight this battle. And I'm sharing our story in hopes that it helps someone else not be too late in helping their child.

CHAPTER TIPS

1. Video games can be addictive. If your child plays excessive amounts of video games and has lost interest in school, sports, or other activities, it is time to take video game addiction seriously.

2. Establish a household rule where no video games are allowed during the week.

3. When you allow your child to play video games, have a strict time limit and make it clear that if they violate it the game will be taken away. When they do violate the rule, which they will, take the game away.

4. Watch for the warning signs. If your child's grades suddenly drop, they lose interest in things, or they become easily irritated, an addiction problem is probably brewing.

5. Follow the rules. If a game is recommended for children ages twelve and older, don't allow your underage child to play that game, regardless of what other parents allow. This is your child, not theirs.

CHAPTER 6

Parenting from a Distance

Whenever I go to a restaurant with my family, I have to quell the urge to jump out of my seat with a bullhorn and shout, "Would everyone please power down your devices and talk to each other!" That's because every time we go out to eat the majority of people, both children and adults, are staring at a tablet or smartphone and not talking to one other. It drives me crazy. When did it become ok to replace our family members and friends with a screen?

At a recent dinner out with my family, I noted that the man sitting at the table to my right was attempting to have a conversation with his wife while her eyes moved back and forth between him and the text chat she was having. The man's wife probably didn't hear a word he said, and he didn't even realize it. To my left was a table of four women and a young girl. Two of the women continuously glanced toward their laps where their smartphones were concealed as they pretended to be interested in the conversation occurring with their friends at the table. The young girl with them had a pair of earbuds in and a tablet in front of her the entire time.

She was hypnotized by the game she was playing. When the waitress placed her entrée in front of her, it took the girl a couple of minutes to realize it had arrived. Finally, there was a couple with two young children sitting directly across from us. Both children were quietly fixated on tablets as the couple enjoyed their "alone" time together without any interruptions from their kids.

My family and I enjoy dining out for two reasons: we love to eat, and we love to be together. Being together means talking, laughing, and communicating with each other, not avoiding each other. Sadly, I can't remember the last time I went to a restaurant where the majority of patrons weren't distracted by their devices. I experienced the worst example of this on a recent vacation with my wife and kids. We arrived at a large, open-air restaurant with hundreds of people, mostly families. When we checked in with the hostess, she said, "Follow me, your table is all the way in the back." It felt like I walked the length of two football fields to get to our table. Every step I took I found myself getting more and more irritated, because at every table I passed, children of all ages were glued to a phone or tablet. I remember wishing I had a box of these books with me; I envisioned myself flinging copies like Frisbees onto each table I passed.

When we were finally seated, I took note of the family sitting next to us, a couple in their thirties with two boys around six and eight years old. The couple was sitting across from each other and their two sons were as well. Both boys had their own tablet and were wearing a big pair of headphones. I kept looking over at their table. I couldn't help myself. I wanted to say something. My wife kept kicking my leg under the table, raising her eyebrows, and giving me that *You'd better stop; you're embarrassing me* look. For the entire hour we dined, there was never one verbal or nonverbal exchange between those parents and their sons. It was as if there was a wall between them and their boys.

See for yourself the next time you dine out. Really take note of the lack of communication and interaction, particularly between parents and their children. Most parents do not realize that this is a problem because they are not properly educated about this topic. Historically, the dinner table has been the ideal place to communicate with our children and get to know what is going on in their lives, but that has changed. According to Norman Herr of California State University at Northridge, the average parent spends just three and a half minutes per week in meaningful conversation with their children.[1] Yes, per *week*! And it doesn't help that many chain restaurants now have tablets built right into the table in front of each seat. Talk about taking away the most important part of dinner—spending time and communicating with the people we love.

Screens have no place at the dinner table. They rob kids of the opportunity to improve communication and language skills. They disconnect families from one another, stripping away the opportunity to enjoy each other's company and learn more about each other. Any time we stick a screen in front of our children during meals, we squander an opportunity to solidify our parent-child bond.

Yes, a quick way to calm down a crying or unruly child is to park them in front of a tablet or television screen; I get it. Occasionally this is fine, but for many parents, it's not just occasional. Devices have become built-in babysitters. The next time you're driving, take a look inside the cars around you, particularly if traffic is moving slowly. You will notice the passengers, and sometimes the drivers, scrolling through their phones. If there are young children in the back seat they will most likely be staring into a screen; in some cases the screens are built right into the headrests. Allowing our children some screen time during long drives is fine, but that's not what I'm referring to. I'm talking about the five-minute rides to school or practice.

The dinner table and car rides are full of potential because they present parents the perfect opportunity to talk to their children about their day, learn what is on their minds, and form deep bonds with them. Yet we are allowing screens to steal this from us. I see it every morning when I am pulling into the high school parking lot. There is always a lot of traffic, as there are over a thousand students and staff all converging at the same time. When I look in my rearview mirror I see the same scene every time—a stressed-out parent driving the car and their teenage son or daughter in the front passenger seat wearing earbuds and peering into their phone. There's no parent-child communication, no connection.

The American Academy of Pediatrics recommends children avoid screens prior to eighteen months old and keep it to only an hour a day up to age five.[2] Yet countless babies and toddlers, as well as teens, stare into these machines for multiple hours a day, seven days a week. It's time to do something about this. We must forgo the screen routines and reclaim our kids.

COACHING DILEMMA

My favorite pastime is baseball. As a child I couldn't get enough of it, and I was talented enough to play for one of the top high school baseball programs in the country and went on to play in college. After my son was born he had a bat in his hand before he knew how to drink from a bottle. For many years I was one of the coaches for his travel baseball team. The team and the families involved were very close; the boys played together for years, starting at age nine. When we traveled to play in tournaments, we would often stay overnight at the same hotel and go out together for meals. The boys usually sat together at one table and the adults at another. The boys were always quite loud and goofy at their table, which was to be expected. But when the boys reached sixth grade, suddenly their table went quiet. Each of the boys had gotten their first smartphone, with the exception of my son. They became mesmerized by the screens in front of them and disengaged from one another.

About halfway through the season I decided I couldn't take it anymore. I could not watch all of these wonderful boys sitting at a table together, opting to play games on their phones instead of talking to each other about school, baseball, and life. At first I didn't think it was my place to say anything to the boys because I'm not their father, but then it hit me—I am their coach. I can tell them what they can or can't do when we are together as a team, whether it's on the field or in a restaurant. So I stood up one night at the table where I was sitting with the other parents, and in my coach's voice I told all of my players to hand their phones over to their parents immediately and start talking to each other again. Much to my surprise, the parents all thanked me for doing this. Not one of them was upset with me. After that, whenever we went out to eat as a team, there were no electronic devices allowed at the tables. And guess what? The boys loved it. They laughed, they goofed around, and they talked. They did what boys were supposed to do.

The message here is simple. Our children need to communicate with other children and us, face-to-face, and they need to do it a lot because it is critical to their social and emotional development. We can no longer just cross our fingers and ignore this important issue. We can no longer allow our children to be disengaged from their peers and us and be pacified by a screen. I'm glad I stood up at that restaurant that night and took care of this situation with my team. I sent a powerful message not only to the boys but also to the parents. So don't be afraid to speak out when you are with your friends and their children. Your friends will thank you for it, and your kids might too.

FAMILY TIME

Over the last few years I've had an incredible number of preteens and teens referred to my private practice because they are struggling with everyday life. I like to meet with the parents first so that I can get a clear picture of the problems their children are experiencing. The problems usually have something to do with anxiety, depression, or behavioral issues, and the cause is usually tied to social media or video games. The stories I hear are unbelievable, like the sixteen-year-old who played a specific video game forty hours a week or the boy who developed a fake identity online and came to believe his own lies. These parents feel helpless and ask me what they can do to help their sons and daughters. The answer that I give them is very simple: *talk to them.*

The atmosphere in today's American household is much different than in previous generations. Not many adults are sitting on their porches during the week, socializing with the neighbors. Few kids are running around the neighborhood playing manhunt, dreading the sound of Mom's voice when she calls them in for dinner. Instead, families are cooped up inside their homes, screens in hand, isolated from each other. If we put hidden cameras in some homes to get a glimpse at the new American family, it would look something like this: moms, dads, and kids are all disconnected from each other and connected to a computer screen, tablet, smartphone, or video game console. Dad might be watching the ball game, Mom might be on the computer, and the kids are texting, playing video games, or spending hours on YouTube and Snapchat. Although these families live under the same roof, they barely know each other.

Think I'm exaggerating? Find me a teenager who is not locked away in their bedroom every night, completely disassociated from the rest of the family. Somehow this has become the norm; I see it every day. But just because it is the norm does not mean that it is normal. Parenting 101 says that a child, no matter what age, should not have any electronics whatsoever in their bedroom. A study recently published in *Pediatric Research* strongly suggests that the placement of the TV has a significant impact on kids' viewing habits and therefore their mental, emotional, and physical well-being.[3] The researchers analyzed data from 1,800 kids at age four and again at age twelve to thirteen. The children who had a television in their bedroom at age four had higher body mass indexes, unhealthier eating habits, and higher levels of emotional distress by age thirteen. They were also more likely to experience depressive symptoms, physical aggression, and lower levels of sociability. Just from having a TV in the bedroom. The study didn't assess the effects of computers and smartphones in the bedroom. Ultimately, the bedroom should be a screen-free zone.

Many of us have ignored this advice because we just didn't understand the dangers. But now we do. More children than ever, particularly teens, are becoming reclusive and barely speak to their parents. Instead they are addicted to their devices and hooked on the attention they get from "friends" online. For many of us, our families are falling apart right in front of our eyes and we don't even realize it's happening. Maybe we, too, are busy attending to our own digital needs and forget that our children need our attention.

Parents, if you take just one thing from everything you've read so far, it's this: *get your kids out of the bedroom and into the family room.* There's a reason why we have "family" rooms and "bed" rooms. One is for spending time with family and the other is for sleeping. And please limit your own media use when you are around your children. Lead by example.

Another study that appeared in *Developmental Science* found that babies and toddlers are negatively impacted by their mother's cell phone use.[4] Fifty infants between seven and twenty-four months were assessed for temperament, exploration, and post-disruption reunion and recovery. The study found that infants were less likely to explore their environment and were more distressed when their mothers were using their phones. The children whose mothers showed a greater habitual use of the phone were slower to recover from their distress when their moms did turn their phones off. In short, much like other forms of maternal withdrawal, mobile device use can negatively impact an infant's social-emotional functioning and parent-child interaction.

There are plenty of other studies that prove how parental screen time can affect children. The takeaway from these studies is that parental screen time often leads to children feeling unimportant later in life and developing emotional disorders. There are also reports of children feeling sad, mad, angry, and lonely when parents use cell phones. Bottom line: our children need us to be present.

According to Common Sense Media, teenagers know there is a problem. They know their phone use causes tension at home. A 2016 survey of 1,240 parents and kids from the same households found that 50 percent of the teens "feel addicted" to mobile devices, and 59 percent of their parents agreed that their kids are addicted. And more than one-third of the families surveyed were concerned about the effects that mobile device use was having on their daily lives, whether it was driving, schoolwork, or at the dinner table. As James Steyer, founder and CEO of Common Sense Media, puts it, "Mobile devices are fundamentally changing how families go about their day-to-day lives."[5]

The key findings from the survey are as follows:

- **Addiction**: One out of every two teens feels addicted to their device, and the majority of parents (59 percent) feel that their kids are addicted.
- **Frequency**: 72 percent of teens and 48 percent of parents feel the need to immediately respond to texts, social media messages, and other notifications. Also, 69 *percent* of parents and 78 percent of teens check their devices at least hourly.

- **Distraction**: 77 percent of parents feel their children get distracted by their devices and don't pay attention when they are together at least a few times per week.
- **Conflict**: One-third of parents and teens say they argue with each other on a daily basis about device use.
- **Risky behavior**: 56 percent of parents admit they check their mobile devices while driving; 51 percent of teens witness this.[6]

Remember the teenage boy I mentioned earlier who had his phone taken away by his parents and then left a suicide note? After it came out during our session that the boy spent pretty much all of his time in his bedroom, I gave the parents some simple advice. I told them to have mandatory family talk time every night. They followed my advice, the boy reluctantly started coming out of his room, and the whole family started to get to know each other. The result? The boy got better.

Our children need us. They need to have conversations with us, and we need to have conversations with them. Think about your own family for a minute and ask yourself the following questions.

- Do you sit down and have meaningful conversations with your children on a daily basis?
- Does your child spend a lot of time in their bedroom alone?
- Do you spend a lot of time, alone, in front of a screen?

How did we get to this point? There are several causes. First, more parents of this generation have a hard time saying no to their children. We fear that saying no is going to harm the relationship we have with them. Next, all of the technology, devices, and screens have made their way into our lives at such a lightning-fast pace that we didn't see it coming. Finally, the addictive nature of screens and devices and the conflicts that ensue have become so common that it almost seems normal. I can assure you it is not normal.

THE DINNER TABLE

In 2014 I was selected to host a television pilot for Food Network called *Can Dinner Save My Family*. The purpose of the show was to transform a family in need by requiring them to commit to having dinner together for thirty straight days. Although Food Network did not develop the pilot into a series, they did air the pilot episode, which focused on a single mother of three who was having a hard time with her troubled fifteen-year-old son. The son had recently been released from a juvenile detention center, and the mother was desperate to repair her relationship with him. I instructed the family to prepare and eat dinner together for thirty straight days. The thirty-day dinner intervention worked for this family; they became closer, argued less, and communicated better.

Studies have shown that children who regularly eat dinner with their families are less likely to engage in risky behavior, less likely to develop mental health disorders, and more likely to do better in school and be happier overall. Unfortunately, many of us are spread so thin between work and chauffeuring our children to activities that we don't have the time to sit together for dinner on a consistent basis or even at all.

Those of us who do sit down for dinner often allow the TV to be on or handheld devices to be used during the meal. One in three adults can't get through a meal without looking at their phone, so it's not just a kid thing.

According to Study Finds, researchers from Nutrisystem polled two thousand adults to determine how distracted we are at the dinner table.[7] Twenty-nine percent of those polled indicated that the phone joined them at every meal, while more than half said they brought their device to the table most of the time. Only 17 percent stated that the phone never came with them to a meal. Although the study was meant to connect poor eating habits and weight gain to the equation, for me it underscored everything I've mentioned thus far about the collapse of the parent/child bond.

The dinner table should be a sacred place. Eating together gives us an opportunity to know what is going on in our children's lives. When television and other screens mix in with dinnertime, the important communication needed by both our children and us is reduced. Start making it a habit to have dinner together most nights of the week and establish a rule that no electronic devices are allowed during family mealtime.

When I was a child, family dinner was mandatory in the Kersting household—every night. My brother and sisters and I had to be at the dinner table every night at 6:00 p.m., no questions asked. Before we ate, we would all hold hands and my father would say grace and give thanks for our wonderful food and family. In today's fast-paced world it can seem impossible to have a set family dinnertime—I get it. But I'm here to tell you that it's not impossible. In my household, we eat together almost every night. My family doesn't have a set time like I did when I was a child, but we still manage dinner. Some nights I don't get home until 8:00 p.m., and although that's late, we still try to eat together because my wife and I know the importance of this ritual. During dinner, no television or electronics are allowed. We talk and we eat. I get to learn about my children's days and they get to learn about mine. But most important of all, we get to know each other and connect with each other because we are disconnected from cyberspace.

CATCHING THE MOMENT

Several years ago I took a trip to an indoor waterpark with my parents, my siblings, and all of our children. My brother and I raced around the park with our boys, hopping from one waterslide to the next. My brother had a waterproof camera with him and was preparing to use it on one of the more popular slides. Right before he was about to go down the slide with his son, he had the camera ready to go. When we met at the bottom of the slide I asked him if he had "caught the moment." He responded, "I certainly did." I then said, "Joe, do you realize that by 'catching the moment' you actually missed the moment?" He looked at me, confused.

Do you miss the moment with your kids? Are you fully immersed in the present moment when you are with them, or are you distracted by your smartphone or computer? If the communication flowing in your home resembles that of the waiting room at your dentist's office, then you are missing the moment with your children. You are missing their growth. You are growing apart from your children, and they are growing apart from you. Your home becomes nothing more than a daily gathering of strangers possessed by a bunch of screens.

Whenever I watch my favorite team, the New York Yankees, on television, I love to observe the fans behind home plate. I notice that many of them aren't actually watching the game. Instead they are taking photos and selfies to show everyone how amazing their seats are and how amazing they are by extension. And if they aren't snapping pictures from their close-up seats, they are texting or using social media while the game is being played. It happens at all sporting events. Just watch an NBA basketball game and pay attention to the fans sitting courtside. Many of them are staring at their phones and missing the game. One clip I saw had me laughing out loud. During a basketball game a loose ball went into the crowd and smacked a woman right in the face because she was watching her phone, not the game. The camera caught the whole moment perfectly. When watched in slow motion, you can see the ball as it hits the woman squarely in the face. Thankfully, she wasn't hurt, but the footage was hysterical. The point I'm making is that we miss many moments, including game-winning shots, because we are either trying to catch the moment on camera or we are distracted.

What's more, our irresistible craving to use our devices, snap pictures, and post things on social media in the moment is not only distracting; it can be downright dangerous and even deadly. According to an August 2018 article in *USA Today*, the world's largest lifeguard organization, the German Lifeguard Association, claims there is a direct link between the risk of children drowning and the smartphones parents hold in their hands.[8] They issued a warning to adults after more than three hundred drownings occurred in the nation in 2018. Peter Harzheim, president of the German federation of swimming pool supervisors, said, "We're experiencing on a daily basis that people treat swimming pools like kindergarten and simply don't pay attention."[9] The article goes on to mention a 2015 incident in which a mother from Texas was charged after a witness claimed she was using her phone while three of her children drowned in an apartment complex pool.

Kidnapping is another potential problem distracted parents may encounter. We remind our children to stay away from strangers and never get into a car with someone they don't know. Yet it is possible that our children can be snatched right from under our noses. Joey Salads is a social experimenter and child safety advocate who uses video to conduct his experiments. His videos receive millions of views on YouTube. One such experiment was for a mother who believed her "phone distracted" husband wasn't paying attention to their son when he took him to the playground. So Joey and the mom decided to do something about it. They arrived at the playground where the dad had taken the boy. They stalked the dad with a hidden camera for a little while and found him sitting on a bench, completely glued to his phone while his son played. You can see this footage on YouTube, but here's what happens: Joey then sneaks over to the bottom of a slide as the young boy comes down it. He offers him some candy, which the boy immediately takes. The boy then follows Joey outside of the playground for some more candy. The father has no idea what is happening because he is too busy staring down at his phone. A little while later the father looks up from his phone and notices that his son is gone. Panic-stricken, he frantically starts searching for his son. Eventually Joey and the mom come out from their secret hiding spot with the boy. The video is a great lesson for parents.

Kidnapping is scary, but the other takeaway from the video is that whenever we are looking at a screen, whether it's because we are trying to capture a moment or because we are distracted, we are not "here" and we miss out on a lot. We miss out on creating real-life memories through our experiences. Our children grow so fast, and before you know it you won't be able to watch them slide down a slide or swing on a swing. So put down the cameras and phones and be in the moment; be in the now.

SCREEN-FREE VACATIONS

Family vacations are great chances to make memories, but they, too, are being invaded by modern technology. If you've been to a resort or hotel pool lately, you'll see that most of the people who are unwinding and catching some rays are totally not "in the moment"; instead they are distracted by their devices. It drives me crazy when I'm vacationing with my family and I see so many kids lying on recliners by the pool playing videos games or watching movies instead of swimming. And I often wonder how many other kids are in their hotel rooms playing on screens instead of playing outside.

According to a *Daily Mail* story, the Wyndham hotel chain knew it had a problem when hotel managers were requesting more beach chairs to accommodate the growing number of guests who would sit and stare at their devices.[10] Wyndham discovered that the average resort guest was bringing three devices to the pool and checking them eighty times a day. They began to offer guests a soft pouch to lock their devices in and include perks for doing so, like free snacks or prime spots around the pool. Wyndham Grand Resorts offer families a 5 percent discount on their stay if they put their phones in a timed lockbox.

Although hotels that limit cell phone use risk losing valuable exposure on social media, along with Wyndham, a growing number of hotel chains are taking the risk. Some resorts now offer such perks as free snorkeling or board games to guests who go phone-free. Many are offering these options because their mission is to promote wellness and relaxation, and screens are getting in the way of this mission.

Other resorts and hotels mentioned in the article have digital-detox concierges who will "cleanse" your suite of all electronics and replace them with board games. At Miraval, a Hyatt-owned resort in Arizona that will be opening additional locations in Texas and Massachusetts, phones are banned in most public places and staff members wear name tags with reminders to unplug and be present. Other resorts encourage a total ban on electronics. Although many of the guests at these resorts embrace the idea of disconnecting, some do not want the plug pulled. Such an inability to disconnect from devices truly validates how serious an issue this is.

The company that manufactures the lock-pouches used by these resorts, Yondr, has a simple purpose: to show people how powerful a moment can be when they aren't documenting or broadcasting it. As people enter a venue, such as a concert hall (or hotel pool area), their phones are placed in Yondr's specialized locking cases. Once attendees enter the phone-free zone, the cases will lock. Attendees maintain possession of their phones but are free to enjoy the event without distraction. If at any point attendees need to use their phone, they simply step outside the phone-free zone and unlock the case. Although famous rock stars and comedians love it, the company has also begun renting its devices to schools, restaurants, wedding venues, sporting events, and hotels. Graham Dugoni, the founder of Yondr, says of his company's mission, "I view it as a social movement, and this is one piece of the puzzle. It's about helping people live in the digital age in a way that doesn't hollow out all of the meaning in your life."[11] It's a great idea and Yondr profits from it, but if we put our minds to it we wouldn't need Yondr cases. All we need to do is to learn a little self-control and teach this to our children.

I'm sharing these examples with you because at every youth game I coach, I notice most parents are distracted by their phones and often miss a lot of what is going on. Yes, they are at the game physically to support their children, but they are not there mentally—they are in another world. Keep this in mind whenever or wherever you are with your kids. If you are in the same room with them or in the bleachers at one of their games and are constantly going back and forth from the task at hand to your phone, you aren't really there. Your children will pick up on this. It sets a bad example and also teaches them that it is ok for them to do the same.

There is nothing in this world more important than our children. They desperately need us to be present and we need them to be present too. My purpose is to raise your level of awareness and understanding. I hope by this point you are ready to make some changes and take some action in order to *reconnect* your family. Below are some tips to make it easier for you.

CHAPTER TIPS

1. Leave your phones in the car when you go out to dinner.

2. Bring some books for your children to read when you are at a restaurant and encourage a lot of verbal communication as well.

3. Establish a rule that there are to be no devices or earbuds allowed during daily car rides with your children. Some screen time is ok for long trips.

4. Practice what you preach. When you are home make sure to spend less time on your own device and more time in person with your family.

5. Try to have uninterrupted dinners together with your family most nights of the week.

6. Never allow screens, including televisions, in your child's bedroom—ever.

7. Be in the moment when you attend your child's events.

CHAPTER 7

How Handheld Devices Impact Emotional Development

Emotional Intelligence (EQ) is the ability to use, understand, and manage emotions in a productive, healthy way. It is what helps us communicate effectively, empathize with others, and overcome life's challenges. Studies have shown that people with high EQs have better mental and physical health, build stronger relationships, and perform better at their jobs. Studies have also shown that a high EQ matters twice as much in terms of superior leadership as IQ does. Unfortunately, emotional intelligence is not something that is taught in the classroom the way that English and history are, even though EQ just may be the most fundamental skill for success.

Dr. Daniel Goleman, a well-known psychologist, has created something known as the "mixed model" for emotional intelligence, which has five key areas:

- **Self-awareness**: Self-awareness involves knowing your feelings, understanding what your emotional triggers are, and knowing how to deal with them.
- **Self-management**: Self-management entails keeping the emotions in check when they become disruptive. It's the ability to prevent outbursts and instead talk calmly during a disagreement.
- **Motivation**: Most people are motivated by outside things like money or other luxuries. Emotionally intelligent people are intrinsically motivated. They know that the outside stuff cannot provide joy and happiness, so that does not motivate them. They are motivated for the sake of joy and productivity.
- **Empathy**: The first three areas involve handling one's own emotions. Empathy, on the other hand, is the ability to support the emotions of someone else. It is the ability to read another person's emotions and respond appropriately.
- **Social skills**: This is the ability to communicate with others. People with strong social skills can find common ground with others at work, school, or anywhere, and have the ability to be persuasive.[1]

Who wouldn't want their children to master these important skills? Unfortunately many twenty-first-century kids can't. Low EQs across the board are the reason why the phone at my private counseling practice is ringing like never before and why there are so many students at my high school having emotional breakdowns. It is also why colleges across the country are seeing double the number of emergency calls to their counseling departments. According to a September

2015 article in *Psychology Today* written by Peter Gray, a research professor at Boston College, students are having emotional crises and are seeking professional help for minor, everyday problems. For example, one student was frantically upset about being called a rude name, and two other students saw a mouse in their apartment and subsequently sought counseling for trauma.[2]

AFRAID TO FAIL

According to Gray, faculty at colleges all across America have noted that students' emotional fragility has become a serious problem when it comes to grading. Some professors have admitted that they are afraid to give low grades for poor performance because of the resulting student meltdowns they would have to deal with in their offices.

Heads of counseling from a group of universities met several times to discuss the lack of student resilience they were experiencing on their campuses, and what these counselors were experiencing is no different from what is being reported across the country with regard to the current mental and emotional states of late adolescents and young adults.

- Students are more needy and less resilient, leading faculty to do more hand-holding, lower academic standards, and not challenge students too much.
- Faculty feel a sense of helplessness, and many members are frustrated with the current situation. However, few had ideas about what institutions could do to address the issue.

- Students are afraid to fail. They do not take risks and need to be certain about things. For many, failure is seen as catastrophic and unacceptable, while external measures of success are seen as more important than learning and autonomous development.
- Faculty, particularly younger members, feel pressured to consent to students' wishes or risk receiving low teaching ratings from their students. For example, students email about inconsequential things and expect rapid responses.
- Students are very uncomfortable about not being right, and want to redo papers to correct mistakes. There is a need for colleges to normalize being wrong, struggling, and learning from one's errors.[3]

Do hours and hours of time spent using social media and technology figure into this dilemma? I believe they do. Remember the multitasking research we discussed in chapter 4? Well, it turns out that the same area of the brain adversely affected by multitasking is also the area responsible for managing emotions. According to researcher Clifford Nass, "A strong emotional intelligence equals a healthy cerebral cortex, the frontal part of the brain that is responsible for executive functions."[4] When a message comes to the brain, it goes first to the amygdala. A brain that is working effectively will then send that message to the cerebral cortex, which decides what to do with the information. People with low emotional intelligence have a weak connection between the emotional part of the brain (the amygdala) and the thinking part of the brain (the cerebral cortex). Think of it this way: they just can't get the right message to the thinking part of their brain. This weak connection leads to a host of different issues such as social anxiety, general anxiety, and depression.

I mentioned that EQ is the ability to regulate one's emotions as well as understand the emotions of others. It is not something we are born with; it is something that can only be learned through observing voices, body posture, and facial expressions. In other words, it can only be learned and developed through face-to-face interaction with other people, not screen-to-screen interaction. The learning starts when we are young and, according to Clifford Nass, it turns out that it is hard. It was easier for previous generations, like mine, to develop strong EQs because communicating face-to-face was all we had. There was nothing else to do. We couldn't whip out a smartphone or tablet to fill our downtime or to communicate with others. Bottom line: if you are distracted, you can't learn, and that includes learning emotions and proper human communication skills.

Campus mental health officials continue to report that students are having a harder time than ever bouncing back from adversity, including common, everyday stressors. Thankfully, colleges are finally taking action to help restore students' resilience and improve their emotional intelligence. For example, many are inviting students to hear about the importance of failure. According to an April 2019 Associated Press article, colleges across America are trying to ease students' anxieties around failure by teaching them to cope with it. Peter Forkner, director of Bentley's counseling center, says, "Failure is normal. It's healthy. And I think people on this panel would argue it actually is transformative. If you're not failing, it probably means you're not taking enough risks."[5]

Some of the interventions highlighted in the article that colleges are offering to fragile students include the following:

- UCLA offers "grit coaching." GRIT stands for guidance, resilience, integrity, and transformation. Any student can enroll in these individualized coaching sessions, which include stress management, time management, communication skills, meditation, mindfulness, cultural humility, goal setting, and more.

- The University of Minnesota hosts a "resilience resource fair" for students interested in mental health, well-being, and resilience.

- Dozens of other schools are now providing "Adulting 101" workshops.

- Stanford University, as part of their resiliency project, offers something called "Stanford, I Screwed Up." This annual event commemorates and celebrates the "epic failures" in our lives. Students can share their failure experiences through storytelling, poetry, video, music, comedy, and more.

- Smith College issues students a "Certificate of Failure." The certificate says, "You are hereby certified to screw up, bomb, or fail at one or more relationships, friendships, text messages, papers, exams, classes, extracurricular activities, or any other choices associated with college . . . and still be a totally worthy, utterly excellent human being."[6]

I'm glad that schools are taking action, but it's also sad that we are at this point. You have to wonder if normalizing failure is the proper way to toughen up kids. Personally I think it's just damage control, but at least it's a start. What we really need to do is understand how our kids got here in the first place so we can prevent similar results in the future. There are many different opinions about the causes, ranging from helicopter parenting to protecting our kids from failure to social media's images of perfection. It is probably a combination of all these things and more, but I do think much of it is related to social media, which encourages everyone, especially young folks, to compare their lives with others'. When everyone else's life seems so perfect, it's easy to feel like a failure. Social media is completely superficial and breeds insecurity.

THE COMPARISON TRAP

How do you think so many college kids got to such a place of insecurity and fear of failure? Think about that for a moment. If everyone else's perfect life and perfect grades and perfect everything is constantly rubbed in your face, aren't you going to compare yourself to them? How can you not become insecure? And it's not just college students experiencing this. Parents are too.

Remember the recent "varsity blues" college admissions bribery scandal that involved Hollywood actresses and other elites? What would motivate someone to pay $500,000 to get their children admitted into a specific university? Is it because this school would provide an opportunity to get a better job that would pay more money? No, money wasn't the issue. The issue was insecurity. This is the ultimate example of, "I need to protect my child from failure," and "I need to protect myself from looking like a failure among my Hollywood friends." These parents, like so many of us, compared themselves to others and needed to come across as successful parents. I'm sure social media had a lot to do with it.

Social media is the ultimate "look at me" platform, and it can be downright dangerous. Think about the message this sends to children: *You're no good so we're going to cheat to make you look good.* That approach will always have the opposite effect because it will only lead to anxiety, insecurity, and self-doubt.

Think I'm exaggerating? According to a 2015 report from the Center of Collegiate Mental Health, the number of college students visiting college counseling centers increased 30 percent between 2009 and 2015.[7] And, according to a survey by the American College Health Association of more than 63,000 college students at 92 schools, 22 percent of college students surveyed in spring 2017 were diagnosed with anxiety or treated for it in the prior year. In the same time period 40 percent of students reported feeling so depressed that they had difficulty functioning.[8]

The mental health issues among college-age students are very real, and our younger children will be there before we know it. A recent study tracked 3,400 tween girls ages eight to twelve, which is the most critical time of development, to look at media use, face-to-face communication, and multitasking. Specific questions were asked with regard to social and emotional development. Those girls who used media while socializing with friends exhibited:

- Fewer feelings of being normal
- Greater feelings of peer pressure

- More friends who were bad influences
- Less sleep[9]

Heavy online media use was also associated with negative social and emotional traits. There was, however, one variable in the study that had a positive predictor of social and emotional development, and it was the amount of face-to-face interaction.[10] Remember the recipe for a strong EQ? That's right, lots of face-to-face communication.

The sharp decrease in emotional well-being is happening at every educational level. My job and my twenty-five years of experience qualify me to tell you that the number and severity of mental and emotional health issues I'm seeing is off the charts. I always tell folks that I wish they could shadow me for a day at the high school or at my private counseling practice. Although the majority of students are functioning well, there is an alarming number who are not. And, yes, they all share one commonality: they are highly immersed in their electronic and social media world. My biggest concern right now is where today's infants and toddlers will be when they are teens. Current research is showing that preschoolers are already developing emotional and behavioral problems because of screen time.

Another recent study has shown that preschoolers who had two hours or more of screen time each day showed clinically significant behavioral problems.[11] When compared with children who had less than thirty minutes per day of screen time, those exposed to more than two hours per day were five times more likely to have behavioral problems and seven times more likely to exhibit traits of ADHD. The study also screened for other problems such as aggression, sleep disturbance, emotional reactivity and anxiety, and depression. According to Sukhpreet Tamana, one of the study's first authors,

> The two big takeaways from this study are that children exposed to more screen time, at either age three or five years, showed significantly greater behavioral and attention problems at age five, and that this association was greater than any other risk factor we assessed, including sleep, parenting stress, and socioeconomic factors.[12]

The researchers in the study concluded by recommending no more than thirty minutes per day of screen time for preschoolers based on the data they collected.

What concerns me the most about this study is that millions of preschool-aged children are likely spending considerably more than two hours per day on screens and are already developing clinically significant problems. What's going to happen to them when they are teenagers or young adults? What will their psychological and emotional well-being look like? What kind of communicators will they be? How will their social skills fare? I'm truly concerned for their welfare, and I'm doing my best to reach parents before it's too late. If you have preschool-aged children, do yourself a favor and listen to the researchers: keep your kids off of screens, get them involved in sports or other activities, and make sure they are spending plenty of time outdoors and interacting with other children.

SOCIAL SKILLS

Several years ago I attended a nice ceremony for my son, who was bridging from Cub Scouts to Boy Scouts. There were a lot of parents in attendance whom I knew well. One particular couple, Christine and Sanj, both cardiologists, were sitting at my table. Christine and I struck up a conversation about the millennial generation and the communication problems they have. Christine works at a university hospital and told me a story about a recent medical school graduate she'd interviewed for a residency. The candidate entered her office, took a seat, and crossed her arms. According to Christine, the candidate looked like she would rather have been watching paint dry than participating in this important interview. As Christine asked her questions, the candidate fidgeted in frustration and answered Christine's questions in a hasty manner. Finally, in a rude way, the candidate said to Christine, "Why are you asking me these questions?" Christine dismissed the candidate and received an impolite, self-absorbed email from her afterward. You would think that someone smart enough to make it through medical school would have the communication skills necessary to do well at an interview, but this young lady clearly lacked emotional intelligence.

For many years I've run a peer leadership program at my high school. During trainings, students are paired with another student from their school. At a recent training, my colleague from another high school nearby, who runs the same program, was short one student, so I sent one of my recruits to his training. When I introduced the two students to each other, there was an awkward silence. Both were really great kids but did not know what to say to each other or even how to look at one another. There was no instinctive introduction, no, "Hello, my name is Joe." And it wasn't the typical shyness you would expect from two fifteen-year-olds; this was outside of the norm. I couldn't help but wonder if their inability to connect with one another was because they'd had so little one-on-one, face-to-face contact in their lives.

I believe that our younger generation is not developing the critical communication and social skills required to ace a job interview or even to simply meet someone new for the first time. As I mentioned when I discussed neuroplasticity, if you don't use a skill you lose the skill. The example of these two students is only one of many. I witness under-developed communication skills every day. After all, as a therapist and counselor, talking to people face-to-face is what I do. Colleagues of mine who are executives are seeing the same thing. They receive stellar résumés from recent college graduates, but when they bring them in for an interview there is something missing. Many of the candidates have a flatness to them, a lack of eye-to-eye transference, and a void of confidence.

Over the years I've noticed more kids having speech problems too. I've hypothesized that the speech issues I've been noticing are because kids are spending way too little time talking face-to-face, which is delaying their speech development. In fact, several speech and language pathologists who have attended my lectures have approached me to let me know that they are dealing with unprecedented levels of speech problems and delays.

Research that was presented at the 2017 Pediatric Academic Societies Meeting suggests that the more time children under the age of two spend playing with handheld screens and devices, the more likely they are to begin talking later and to have delays in expressive speech.[13] Researchers also found that for every thirty-minute increase in handheld screen time, there was a 49 percent increased risk of expressive speech delay. Early language delays are linked to future academic problems and difficulty finishing high school.[14] Children with difficulty expressing themselves are often frustrated, display attention-seeking behavior, and act out.

We need to engage our younger generation, our own children, face-to-face, on a daily basis so that they can develop these important skills. We must push our children and their friends to be mentally and physically present with one another. That means that if your child has a friend over, limit the time spent in front of screens and increase the time spent playing and talking. The more they are exposed to this type of interaction, the stronger their communication skills and emotional intelligence will become.

CHAPTER TIPS

1. Human beings are social/emotional beings. We are wired to communicate with each other face-to-face. Ensure that your child is getting more face-to-face time than screen time.

2. If your child has friends at the house, collect all devices and encourage them to go outside and play.

3. Allow your child to fail. That's right, you heard me. Insulating our children from adversity prevents them from learning and growing. It damages their EQ.

4. Limit your infant or toddler to *zero* minutes of screen time per day. If you hand your child your phone while

shopping or doing something else, you may be harming their emotional and social development.

5. Teach your children to look people in the eye when they speak. This is an important part of communication and a catalyst for social confidence.

CHAPTER 8

The Digital Classroom

How Tech Impacts Learning

In 2008 a sixteen-year-old client I'd been seeing at my private counseling practice showed up with a briefcase. I had been meeting with this boy every week right after school, and this was the first time he'd brought a briefcase instead of his usual backpack. When I asked him why he had a briefcase, he responded, "Oh, it's not a briefcase; it's a laptop case for my new laptop. The school gave it to me." "The school gave you a laptop?" I asked. He responded, "Yes, they gave every student in my school one." At first, this struck me as being pretty cool. At the time technology and computers were nothing new for schools, but giving each student their own laptop was something else.

Today, just about every school district near me provides students with their own personal device, either a laptop or a tablet. It is known as "one-to-one computing" and countless schools throughout the country have adopted this practice, including middle schools. Schools that are not "one-to-one" often use "cows," or computers on wheels, which is basically a cart that holds a bunch of computers and can easily be transported from room to room. The big question is this: Is computer-based learning a good thing or a bad thing? That depends on who you talk to. I lean toward the latter, because although computers and technology offer some great things, there's still no evidence that computer-based learning improves learning, performance, or grades. In fact, there is evidence that the opposite is true.

Let's dive into this topic a little deeper, so you can decide for yourself whether or not computer-based learning is as innovative and necessary as the tech industry will tell you it is. Is it making our kids smarter?

NOT SO GREAT?

There's a lot of research that shows kids learn and perform better when there's a pen or pencil in hand rather than a keyboard. Additionally, most of the teachers I've spoken with say that computers and tablets pose more of a problem than a benefit because they distract the students. And parents are caught in the middle. During the Q&A part of my lectures, for example, parents will always ask me how they are supposed to curb their child's screen time if the school gives them a computer that they are required to use. Great question, complicated answer.

I haven't met a parent yet who has raised their hand or approached me at a lecture to tell me that computers and technology are the greatest thing that's ever happened to their child academically. And I've never had a parent at my high school say anything positive about computer-based learning—but they complain about it a lot.

As schools adopt curricula that use more technology, teachers have more opportunities to utilize new and different teaching methods that are more compatible to modern-day, digital-native learners. Or so we're told. The resources are out there in the form of tools, apps, e-textbooks, and even gaming that is educational in nature. These resources are intended to enhance learning and make it more fun. Students now have instant access to any research or resources they need. They can work more effectively with their peers and easily share information. All of this sounds impressive, but teachers aren't totally sold on it. Most teachers I've met with say that although computers offer some benefits, they also perpetuate cheating and distractibility. Student engagement is also lessened because teachers now have to compete against computers and phones for students' attention.

Last school year, a history teacher I've known for many years came to my office to discuss one of her students. She's the most passionate teacher I've ever worked with; she lives and breathes teaching. During our conversation, the topic of computers and devices came up. She said, "Tom, I have twenty-four students in my class and only three of them are learning; the rest cannot stop looking at their computers or phones. I've tried disciplining them but it takes up the entire class time. All I can do is focus on the ones who want to learn, and I am beyond frustrated." She then began to cry. Thankfully, she has initiated some new rules in her classroom this year. She now has a shoe holder hanging on the wall in her classroom; students are required to place their phones in a shoe slot when they arrive. She also doesn't allow students to have their laptops open when she is lecturing, and she tries to minimize the amount of computer-based assignments in the classroom.

According to a 2015 report by the Organization for Economic Cooperation and Development (OECD), "In countries where it is more common for students to use the internet at school for schoolwork, students' performance in reading declined between 2000 and 2012, on average."[1] The results from this report also showed no appreciable improvements in student achievement in reading, mathematics, or science in countries that had invested heavily in information and communication technologies. According to a 2018 *Guardian* article, the journal *Frontiers in Psychology* identifies an absence of research supporting the enthusiastic claims that tablets will "revolutionise education."[2] The author explains that technology in education is often justified on the grounds that it boosts disadvantaged children, even though research shows it widens socioeconomic divides rather than bridging them. One of the biggest initiatives to date has been the "One Laptop per Child Programme," which distributed twenty-five million low-cost computers with learning software to children in the developing world. However, the initiative failed to improve language or math results.[3]

Remember the large experiment conducted at West Point to see how classroom computing affected learning? The students who were allowed to use a laptop to take notes in class did significantly worse on the final exam than students who did not use laptops. A Canadian study on e-learning similarly found that students don't really like e-learning all that much; they prefer a smart person in the front of the room teaching them real life lessons.[4]

BIG TECH

If there's no research suggesting that computer-based learning is any better than traditional learning, and parents, students, and teachers aren't sold on it, why is it taking over our schools? In a May 2017 special report that appeared in *Edweek Market Brief*, editor Sean Cavanagh explains how the three major tech companies, along with relative newcomer Amazon, are going head-to-head in vying for big chunks of school business mainly through the sales of devices and operating systems. Even though these companies are known more for their work outside of education, they are now making a fortune in the education sector. Their vendors are learning what schools want and are dazzling administrators and students with their products. To date, Google has carved out the biggest slice of the education pie thanks to the simplicity and cost-effectiveness of its Chromebook. In response, Microsoft, which has long been a leading producer of operating systems, has created a new operating system with a set of classroom tools to compete with Google's G Suite for education. Apple's devices are also used in schools, with tools that are more focused on coding, music, and video. Finally, newbie Amazon offers its Amazon Web Services, which many schools use for cloud-based storage.[5]

Cavanagh goes on to detail how these big tech companies are spending a lot of money in the education market to improve their market share. For example, Google gives its G Suite operating system to schools for free because they're investing in the millions of children walking through the school doors every day, luring them into their brand and creating brand loyalty. They are essentially "seeding for future revenue." Customers for life—it's brilliant. In 2014 Google faced public criticism after a class action suit was brought against them for data-privacy practices. Google admitted to scanning and indexing email messages from millions of students through its G Suite. Google has since signed a student privacy pledge agreeing not to sell students' personal information or build profiles of students that could be sold to advertisers.

That's progress in the moral realm, but are the tools actually effective in the classroom? According to Hal Friedlander, former chief information officer for New York City Public Schools,

> While Apple, Google, and Microsoft have developed good products that they sincerely believe meet students' and teachers' needs, their products are falling well short of transforming teaching and learning. Innovation has suffered. The products turned out by the major tech companies do not amount to groundbreaking stuff that propels teaching into some new realm because of the technology.[6]

In 2017 the *New York Times* did a great piece about the way tech companies use schools to promote their products.[7] The article compared the tech industry's methods for pushing its products in schools to those methods mastered by the pharmaceutical industry. Drug companies regularly pay doctors to give speeches and offer them free meals because these perks influence prescribing practices. Tech companies have gone as far as flying school officials to speak at events and often take them to expensive restaurants in an effort to influence them to purchase their products. Rob Reich, a Stanford political science professor, called it a "pay-for-play" arrangement.[8]

Dallas Dance, former superintendent of the Baltimore County Public Schools, was particularly scrutinized. Dance was quoted as saying that every school must provide an equitable digital learning environment—including giving every student a device, including first graders. His district awarded Daly Computers with a $205 million contract to furnish an HP device known as the Elitebook Revolve for every student. Soon after the deal was done, HP invited Dance to give a keynote speech at a major education conference in New York. Dance then appeared in an HP video, and his school district received a "visionary award" from Microsoft, the company that owns the software that runs the laptops. All told, between March 2014, when the laptop contract was announced, and April 2017, when Dance retired, he had taken sixty-five out-of-state trips related to his school district's tech initiative, costing the district more than $33,000.[9]

The *New York Times* piece concluded its investigation by covering Baltimore County Public Schools' 2017 fundraising luncheon, which was arranged by its educational foundation. Tech companies made significant donations, and some of their directors even sat on the foundation's board. Of course Daly Computers was the biggest donor, giving $30,000. Of the $211,500 in donations that the event raised, 43 percent of it came from tech companies. According to Michael Collins, a former Maryland senator and school board member, "You have all these huge contracts, and then you donate all this money, and the foundation puts up a banner advertising your company's name; I just don't think it passes the smell test."[10]

FUELING ADDICTION

Although ethics comes into question when school officials and big tech partner up, there's a bigger issue that I don't think school officials have given enough thought to: addiction. Now that gaming disorder is officially a diagnosable disease, the door is wide open for other technology addiction diagnoses. Screen addiction disorder is already being considered for further review by the American Psychological Association. If the APA or the WHO adds this to their list of diagnosable diseases, how are schools going to handle screen usage and distribution? I can make the argument that more than half of all kids right now would fit the diagnosis of "screen addicted." Suppose that five years from now half of all kids actually have the diagnosis? What are schools going to do if half of its students have doctor's notes saying that they cannot use any type of screen for learning? Will schools be prepared for this? Can they adjust?

Countless parents have told me that their children are completely addicted to screens and that the school-issued computers their children are required to use to complete assignments aren't helping. Their children simply cannot control themselves from drifting off to social media, games, or YouTube. Some parents I've communicated with have already started showing up to the main offices of their child's school with the laptop in hand, basically saying, "Take this thing and shove it; figure out another way to teach my kid."

Schools are becoming too reliant on computers. Either they find a balance, or I predict that they're going to have their hands full with fed-up parents in the coming years. Schools will need to be more proactive today in order to prepare for tomorrow. Perhaps they should contact the Waldorf School in Silicon Valley for some advice. In this school, where 70 percent of the students enrolled are sons and daughters of Silicon Valley tech executives, you won't find a screen anywhere. They take a more holistic approach and believe in the role of the imagination and intellect by integrating creative development into student learning. Remember, these are the children of the people who are developing all the screens. Could there be something these Silicon Valley tech executives know that others don't?

CHAPTER TIPS

1. If your child seems addicted to their laptop or tablet, and they are required to use it for school assignments, contact the school and request paper and pen assignments.

2. If your child's school is a "one-to-one" school, and the school-issued laptop is causing more harm for your child than good, turn in the device and insist that the school find a more traditional way to educate your child.

3. Do your best to ensure that your child's school-issued device has social media sites blocked. Talk to school officials to ensure this.

4. Make sure your child does homework in a central location, like the kitchen. They are less likely to wander onto social media, YouTube, or video games if they know you are in the vicinity.

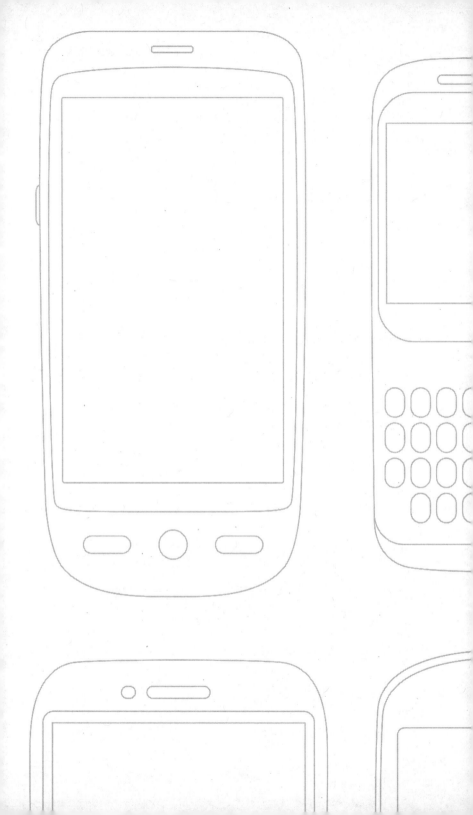

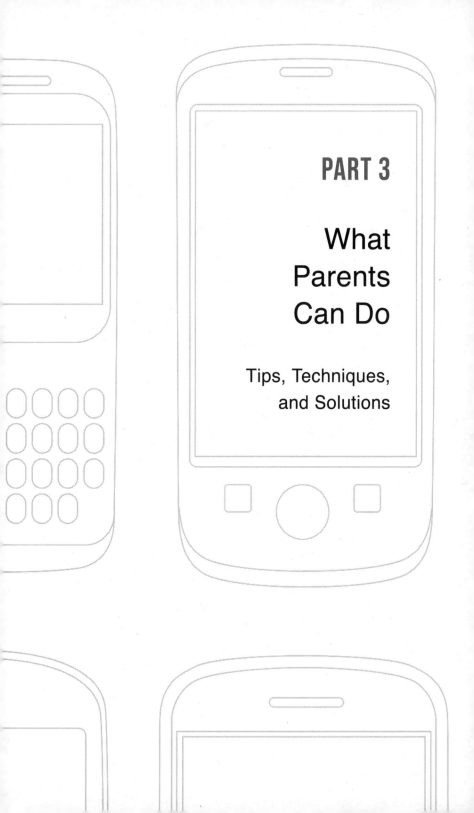

PART 3

What Parents Can Do

Tips, Techniques, and Solutions

CHAPTER 9

Raising Our Children to Be Leaders Instead of Followers

As I'm writing this my daughter is twelve years old and in the sixth grade. She's one of only a handful of children in her grade without a phone. Most of her classmates bring a phone to school with them and are already marinating in Snapchat and Instagram before their classes even start. Here's a crazy fact that bears repeating: the average age of first smartphone issuance is now 10.3 years old. It's already mainstream. There's rarely a day that my daughter doesn't ask me for a phone. This has caused conflict between us because she thinks I am being too strict, and she feels left out. I understand how she feels, and I feel bad about it, but I'm hoping one day she'll understand. I tell her to trust me. There's a saying my father used to use that has always stuck with me. It goes like this: God didn't give you to me for me to trust you; he gave you to me for you to trust me.

There's typically anywhere from a hundred to five hundred parents in attendance at my lectures. To keep everyone's attention, I capitalize on humor and audience participation. For example, I will say to the audience, "Please raise your hand if you think it is appropriate for your middle school child to have M-rated video games like *Call of Duty* or *Grand Theft Auto*." As expected, not a single hand goes up; everyone agrees it's a terrible idea. Next, I say, "Please raise your hand if your child has one of these games." Again, not a single hand is raised, but I notice a lot of fidgeting and uncomfortable body language. Then I say, "Ok, so everyone agrees that M-rated games are not good for children under eighteen and no one in this room should allow their children to have them. But the statistical truth is that more than half of you in attendance do allow your children to play and own these games. In fact, you're the one who bought it for them. So more than half of this room is not being very truthful." I try not to put anyone on the spot or make anyone feel uncomfortable. I'm just trying to help people understand their own behavior. This dialogue with parents about M-rated games is a lead-in to my next topic, which is something known as social conformity.

FOLLOW OR LEAD?

Conformity is a type of social influence involving a change in belief or behavior in order to fit in with a group. Let's say your son is in fourth grade, around ten years old. You have always told him that he is not allowed to play M-rated video games until he is eighteen, and you were firm about this because you are a responsible parent. Then Christmas comes and one of your son's good friends gets *Call of Duty* as a gift. Before long all of your son's friends get the game. You start to feel bad for your son because he is the only one whose parents won't break the rules and allow him to have this game. You go back and forth in your mind trying to figure out what you should do. Finally, you say to yourself, *You know what, every other kid has the game; the boys are now eleven, and they are a little more mature. If all of the other parents are ok with it, I guess it must not be that big of a deal. Plus, I want him to fit in, I don't want him to feel left out, and I certainly don't want him to get picked on for being the only kid who is not allowed to have these games. What the heck, he's doing well in school and he's responsible—I guess it's not a big deal.* And so you get your son *Call of Duty* for his birthday.

This is a classic example of social conformity or peer pressure. And yes, it happens to us adults. The problem with this kind of adult peer pressure, this conformity, is that our children learn from us; they model our behavior. When we give in, we teach them to give in. When we ensure that they fit in with everyone else, that they follow suit, we are unintentionally teaching them how to be followers instead of strong leaders.

My daughter doesn't have a smartphone because she's not ready for one. She's not mature enough to handle all that comes with having one. I don't think any twelve-year-old is. Plus, I'd like to believe that her phone-free childhood will underline that the Kerstings don't follow the crowd. I hope that through this experience she will develop strong leadership qualities as she grows up.

A common fear many of us share is that our children won't fit in. And in most cases that's exactly what this feeling is—a *fear*, not a reality. Sometimes we go to the ends of the earth to make sure our children are included in every activity so they don't become irrelevant. I witness this all the time in my community with sports, clothing, and electronic devices. We see what everyone else is doing, and our mind tells us that must be the way to go. Without realizing it, we allow the collective group to make our decisions for us instead of deciding for ourselves what is right for our children. This is why so many younger children now own smartphones. Although they appear to make our children fit in, I believe the risks are too great. The best bit of advice I can give you is to follow your parental instincts and be aware of trends going on around you. If your parental instinct is to tell your child, "Sorry, just because your friends have smartphones doesn't mean that you should have one," then go with that instinct. You'll be sending your child a strong message, even though they might not understand it now.

Perhaps the most important message I'm trying to convey is that we don't want to teach our children to be followers of the crowd; we want to teach them to be leaders. When we allow our children to have something that we know they are not mature enough to handle, for the sake of fitting in, we are teaching our children to follow the crowd. It is our job as parents to do what is right for our children, not to allow outside influences to decide that for us.

When I have these conversations with parents they sometimes become defensive, because no adult wants to admit they were peer-pressured into anything. A common reaction I get from parents who attend my lectures is that if their child didn't have a smartphone with texting and social media, then their child would have no friends. I understand this rationale and admit that I worried about this too when my son was younger. Now that he is sixteen, I can tell you this was an irrational worry. Even though my son has a phone now, he has never used social media of any kind. He does not have Snapchat or Instagram—and he does not feel that he has missed out on anything. Instead, he is still running around with friends having fun, excelling in school, playing sports, getting plenty of sleep, and simply enjoying being a teenager. The things he's missed out on are the things I want him to miss: gossip, fake news, inappropriate posts, sleep deprivation, fear mongering, and a potentially weakened sense of self. Ignorance is bliss! In fact, I was talking about this with a friend of mine recently, and I told him that if I had gotten my son a smartphone when he was younger, I could say goodbye to his hard work in school, his dedication to sports, and his Eagle Scout aspirations. He likely would have become too distracted by all of the superficial stuff. It is not a trade I was willing to make.

MAKING THE CHOICE

So, let's ask the obvious question: What is the right age to get your child a smartphone? The best answer to this question I have ever heard goes like this: *When you feel comfortable with your child watching pornography.*

If you believe for a second that your child isn't going to click on the provocative images that pop up on a social media site, I want to offer you a reality check. Your child is a great kid. But even great kids can't hold up against a 24/7 temptation. And when they do click on that image, it will take them to places no parent would want their child to go. Are you willing to make that sacrifice? I understand that children have laptops and tablets where inappropriate content can also be accessed, but at least these devices are easier to manage. Smartphones in pockets go with them wherever they go.

In light of all these risks, what will you and your family do? Mark Little, founder and president of Diversified Funding, a leading financial services firm, said it best:

> A leader is someone [who] leads by example and has the integrity to do the right thing even when it is not popular. A good leader has positive influence over others, inspiring them to become a better person and example for others to model their life against, as well.[1]

Our children should memorize this quote and program it into their minds. Kids who have been taught to do what is right and follow the rules become intrinsically guided by their inner character and integrity. Popularity is not on their radar. Their confidence and character are such that even if a peer were to make fun of them for not being part of the social norm, it would be no big deal. Leaders have no face to save and nothing to prove to anyone but themselves.

As parents, we are the only ones who can cultivate character and leadership in our children. I'm not saying any of this is easy; it certainly hasn't been for me, but there is something you can do right now to create change and foster leadership. It's called the Phone Free School Zone Pledge, and it is super simple.

Here is an email from a parent who attended one of my recent lectures. You'll see how simple it is to get started.

Mr. Kersting:

I attended your talk at Bethlehem High School a few weeks ago. I thought it was fantastic, and I loved your suggestion that families and schools work together when children are in the early grades to get a petition going whereby parents would agree to hold off on giving their kids smartphones and access to social media until some later age (like eighth grade or high school).

My daughter is in first grade, and the day after your talk I contacted her principal (who was also at your talk) about how we could implement your phone pledge. She was very supportive, and we are meeting this afternoon to discuss the best way to go about this. I was wondering if you could send me some sample petitions from other districts to look at or if you knew of a parent who helped launch this in another school I could contact with questions.

Also, I'm wondering what you would suggest we have in the petition as the appropriate age for a smartphone/social media.

Thank you for taking the time to come to our town. The work you are doing is so important and really gave my husband and me the confidence we needed to stand firm on these issues.

Best,
Cate C.

FOR OLDER CHILDREN

The Phone Free School Zone Pledge is a prevention tool. It will not work for everyone, of course, but it is a start. It is also not something that can be easily initiated in middle schools and high schools since those kids are already fully immersed in their phones. That doesn't mean it's too late to take action

PHONE FREE SCHOOL ZONE PLEDGE

A phoneless child is a happier child. A happier child is a smarter child. —Tom Kersting

PARENTS . . . TAKE THE PLEDGE!

Do you want your child to be happier, more social, and perform better in school? Did you know that delaying the purchase of a smartphone for your child will improve every aspect of your child's life?

Many parents purchase phones for their children even though they know they aren't ready—and the reason is everyone else does; we fear that our child will be left out. But there's an easy way to reverse unhealthy social conformity and create a healthier one, a PHONE FREE one. It's simple. It's called the *Phone Free Pledge*. All you have to do is sign it while your child is still young and few children of their age have phones; I can't imagine any parent with young children not agreeing to this.

Once the majority of parents in your community sign, a new, healthy social norm will be established, one where parents all agree to delay purchasing phones for their children until late adolescence. There will be no pressure. Your child won't want what nobody else has; that's how kids are wired.

Are you ready to take part in the *Phone Free Pledge*? If so, here's what you can expect from your child:

- Less distractions at school and home
- Improved focus
- Enhanced communication skills
- Avoidance of dangerous social media sites and predators
- A leadership mentality

- Improved relationship with parents and less arguing and bickering over device use
- Enriched family/school relationships
- Less likelihood of developing anxiety and depression
- Less likelihood of harming oneself
- Fewer visits to the nurse's office
- Improved learning
- Better sleep, which improves school performance and mood
- Less bullying, as most bullying takes place through text messaging and/or social media

SCHOOLS . . . ACCEPT THE PLEDGE!

Want to help create a Phone Free School Zone? The best way to get this going is through your local school administration. Your child's school can include the pledge in its summer packet and distribute it to every family with children from third grade down to kindergarten. The petition simply says, "I agree not to purchase a smartphone for my child until late adolescence." It's that simple. All you have to do is check off yes or no. I'm betting that most parents will check YES. What parent wouldn't? Schools will definitely want to be on board as well, because the leading cause of most of the problems they are dealing with is tied to smartphones and social media.

A school that is phone free will:

- Have fewer student suspensions and detentions
- Improve teacher confidence and morale, as students will be more eager to learn and less distracted
- Enrich student learning
- Improve test scores

- Improve the overall mental health of students
- Organically foster an environment where students can become better communicators and develop excellent social/interpersonal skills
- Reduce the diagnoses of ADHD and keep down special education costs
- Improve student confidence and cultivate emotional intelligence

Once schools have secured signatures from parents, the school can send out periodic Phone Free School Zone reminders in the form of tips and other valuable information. This will help keep the parent pledge fresh in everyone's mind, stimulate conversations about it in your community, and begin to foster school and household environments that are phone free.

Think about it! When the majority of parents are on the same page, the pressure to purchase a phone for younger children will be minimal. As your child moves through elementary and middle school, they won't experience any pressure because most of their peers won't have phones either.

The ultimate goal for the Phone Free School Zone initiative is to create a new, healthy social conformity, one where nobody will want smartphones because no one else has them. You can download the petition by going to my website, www.tomkersting.com. Print it and bring it to your school administrators. Make this happen!

SAMPLE PHONE FREE SCHOOL ZONE PLEDGE

I _____ agree to take the pledge. I agree not to purchase a smartphone for my child _____ until late adolescence.

to help these kids. I will never accept that it is too late to do anything. It's never too late to change. The best advice I can give you if you have older children is to start making small changes at home right away. Yes, your child will give you a hard time with any changes you enforce, but they will thank you later on. Here are some simple strategies you can start with.

Strategies for Parents of Middle School Students

- If your child brings a phone to school, starting today your child is no longer allowed to. You will need to step up to the plate and explain to your child that you are the parent, you are in charge, and a phone in school is nothing but a distraction.

- If you are afraid of sending your child to school without a phone because of the possibility of an emergency, read the next chapter carefully; you'll see that most of your fears are unwarranted.

- Do not allow your middle school child to use the device in their bedroom. If your child already does, then make a new rule right away. Remember, you're in charge. You're the parent.

- Be wary of your own device use. You want to lead by example.

- Make your child spend more time with you. Be creative. Bake with your child. Do yardwork with your child. Play catch with your child. Bottom line—be active with your child and make it fun. Don't take no for an answer. Anytime you engage in these types of activities you are pulling your child and yourself away from devices.

- If you purchase a smartphone for your child, make it clear that social media is not allowed. Check the phone regularly.
- Set up a smartphone contract. There's one you can download at my website, www.tomkersting.com.

Strategies for Parents of High School Students

- Make sure your teenager's phone is in a different room when they are doing homework.
- Have a sit-down family meeting and explain that starting right away phones are to be turned in to you at a certain time every night, preferably an hour before bedtime. If your teenager refuses to follow the rules, then it's time for you to get tough and disconnect their phone. After all, you probably pay for it.
- Encourage your teen to read this book.
- Purchase a phone lockbox if necessary. There are many "unplug boxes" you can buy that have timers, making it impossible for your teen to open. Consider putting your phone in the box too.
- Organize more outdoor activities with your family such as hiking and biking. If your teen gives you a hard time, explain the importance of unplugging and spending time in nature. If your teen won't budge, take the phone, TV remotes, and gaming remotes with you on your outdoor excursion. Put everything, including the wireless router, in the trunk of the car, and leave your teen at home without any electronic stimuli.
- Play board games, often.

- If you are constantly tiptoeing around your teen and your teen is calling the shots, this is not just about electronics. You are the parent in your family. You need to roll up your sleeves, take action, and take back control of your home. It's time for some tough love, which may be painful but is necessary. One of the best quotes I've ever heard is, "If your teen doesn't hate you then you're doing something wrong."

We want to raise our children to be leaders, which is difficult to do in this day and age. It is our job to teach our children what leadership is about, and the best way to do that is by example. When we lead by example we are helping them develop exemplary leadership qualities. Your child will fight you tooth and nail to have what everyone else has; it is up to you to decide what is appropriate for your child. If all of your child's friends have phones and yours doesn't because you believe your child is not ready, go with your gut instinct; don't cave in to the pressure to conform.

CHAPTER TIPS

1. Never do what everyone else does simply because everyone else is doing it.
2. Always listen to your instincts. If your gut tells you not to allow your son or daughter to visit a certain website or play a particular game, then don't allow it.
3. If you fear that your child will fade into irrelevancy and you strive to ensure they fit in like everyone else,

you are teaching them to be ordinary. Teach uniqueness and let your children grow from that.

4. Your child will nag you for certain things, so stay firm; don't give in.

5. *No* is the most important word in the parental vocabulary.

6. Have constant conversations with your children about leadership, ethics, and values, starting at a young age.

7. Tell your children you love them—often.

8. You are your child's parent, not their friend.

CHAPTER 10

Fragile Kids

The Media's Impact and
What We Can Do about It

In October 2012 there was a rash of kidnapping attempts throughout my community. Almost daily there was a story of another attempt to lure a child plastered on the cover of every local and regional newspaper. It became the hot topic for the local television news stations too, and everyone's Facebook feeds were blowing up with this frightening news. Everyone around town was talking about the kidnapping attempts, whether at church, at the ball field, or at school. Everyone was on edge. After the nineteenth kidnapping attempt over the span of three weeks, I received a call from a local newspaper reporter asking for my professional insight and advice on this frightening situation. The reporter was stunned by my response because I told her that I didn't think a kidnapper existed. I said to her, "You mean to tell me that the alleged 'kidnapper' failed all nineteen times in their attempt to abduct a child?" Then I gave my version of what I believed was happening. It looked something like this:

> What I believe has happened is that the first luring attempt probably wasn't a luring attempt at all. It was likely a couple of high school boys driving down a street who saw a younger child walking home from school, and they decided to do what many foolish teenagers do, pull a prank. Because teenage boys will be teenage boys, they thought it would be funny to pull their car near the young child and say something like, "Hey, little girl, want some candy?" With that, the well-versed youngster surely sprinted home as fast as she could to tell her mom what had happened, because, like most little girls and boys in the world, she had been taught by her parents to do that. The first thing the girl's mother did was contact the police. And the second thing? She immediately alerted all of her friends on Facebook.
>
> Within minutes, all of the other Facebook moms reposted this RED ALERT message to their friends, and it immediately spread like wildfire. "There is now a kidnapper lurking in our community." Every mom and dad then panicked, and their fear was quickly projected upon their children. Every child in the community became on edge, and they were all talking about it at school. School administrators and teachers were notified and had to come up with a plan. They held an emergency meeting with students the following morning, advising them not to talk to strangers and to be alert. The anxiety among the kids went viral.
>
> Over the ensuing days, a child stopped at the local candy store after school for a treat and noticed a "strange-looking man" parked in the lot. The man signaled to the child, perhaps asking for directions because he was lost, but the paranoid child didn't see it that way; instead he panicked. He

ran home to tell his mom that "the kidnapper" had tried to abduct him. Now that kidnapping attempt number two had occurred, Facebook feeds lit up even more, and the local news salivated. This continued for the next few weeks until now, when there have been nineteen "attempted abductions" in the area.

When I hung up the phone with the reporter I was certain she would not use my comments, and I was fine with that. But my version of the kidnapping attempts was probably right. The following day the great state of New Jersey, my state, was hit with the biggest hurricane in its history, Hurricane Sandy. Thousands of people lost their homes. Millions more lost power for days or weeks. There was chaos throughout the state, and the story lit up the news stations. Hurricane Sandy took over the television screens, computer screens, social media, and newspapers. The "kidnapper" mysteriously disappeared—and not another word was ever mentioned about him. Maybe he got blown away by the fierce winds of Hurricane Sandy.

We are living in fear, and we are projecting this fear upon our children without even realizing it. A breaking news story from the other side of the country will appear on your computer or smartphone screen within seconds. Ten or twenty years ago, we did not have this capability, so if there was a kidnapping in rural Mississippi, for example, we didn't know about it, let alone have the story transmitted to our suggestible brains over and over again.

Our society has changed so drastically because there is just too much *news*. We soak in it because we bring our handheld news-delivery devices with us everywhere we go, including bed. The news organizations love it. They've gone from organizations providing information to organizations battling for people's round-the-clock attention. In the past we would just read the news and go about our day. Now we participate in it through social media, which can virally spread the fear and anger. I believe this overload of information leads to drastic and unnecessary action.

This is why games like dodgeball and tag become banned from school playgrounds after some parent decides to sue the school because their child sprains an ankle or suffers "emotional harm" because they weren't very good at dodging. A story like this can go viral and appear on our phones and TV screens, and *bam*—the game is now banned on playgrounds across the nation. For example:

- A parent of a college freshman sued his son's high school basketball coach and the school because his son did not get enough playing time senior year in high school, and the parent claims he lost out on scholarship money because of it.
- A school district banned "unsupervised cartwheels" during recess after a girl sprained her ankle.
- A liberal arts college in New England banned "booing" at sporting events.[1]

We hear about stories like this because of the incredible reach of digital media, which can prompt other people and school personnel to establish similar extraordinary rules. Just look at the countless schools across the country that have banned kids from playing the harmless game of tag. It started with one news story that went viral and became contagious. How do we avoid this mentality? The tips at the end of this chapter will help prevent you and your children from falling into the "news" trap and becoming overly sensitive and anxious, but first, let's talk about something else we're always anxious about—the threat of an emergency.

IN CASE OF EMERGENCY?

At a lecture I gave a few years ago I shared with the audience that my son and daughter did not have cell phones and were perfectly fine without them. I explained that I did not want my kids' brains bombarded with drama, fake stories, and other mind-altering content; I just wanted them to be kids. One surprised parent asked me how I could live not knowing what my kids were doing or where they were. She asked me, "What if there is an emergency?" I explained to her that every school these days has emergency protocols for everything from serious emergencies like school shootings to routine student health issues. Lockdowns are enforced and lockdown practice drills are regularly mandated by law. A smartphone will not help. For other emergencies such as family emergencies, a simple phone call to the school office will do the trick. School administrators will immediately attend to your needs and gather your child from the classroom. The real issue is that parents have become so dependent on these devices that they now act as a tether keeping our children within arm's reach at all times, and it's not healthy. How can we expect our children to detach from us, spread their wings, and make it as adults if the underlying message that we send to them is that the world is a dangerous place?

Other parents at my lectures have a different take. I will tell stories of students who are distracted all day long, during class, by their cell phones, and some parents will ask, "Then why doesn't the school just ban them from being in the building?" Unfortunately, this is much easier said than done. Furthermore, it is not the school that purchased the phone for the child and is sending them to school with it.

Cell phones entering schools often have very little to do with the school. If a school superintendent sent home a letter notifying parents that students were no longer allowed to bring these devices to school, the school would potentially be hit with lawsuits. Many parents couldn't fathom not being able to get in contact with their child at a moment's notice. In many ways I understand this because of the mass tragedies like those in Columbine and Newtown. However, parents are communicating with their children even when there isn't an emergency or an important change of plans. Often when I call a student out of class whom I need to speak with, during their time with me they will receive text messages from their mom or dad. Keep in mind that their parents don't know their child is with me; they think they are in math or English class, yet they still send their children text messages. Ultimately, cell phones have redefined convenience, and we have become accustomed to being able to reach out to our children and others at a moment's notice. We have become an instant gratification nation, even in our relationships with each other, and in many ways this is not a good thing.

THE ICONNECTED PARENT

In 2011, a book written by Middlebury College professor Barbara Hofer revealed the shocking truth about the overly connected parent/college student relationship. According to Hofer, until recently students handled college on their own, learning life's lessons and growing up in the process. Now students turn to their parents for answers to everything, rendering many of them incapable of learning how to handle life's challenges, like how to turn on an unfamiliar washing machine. Some parents are so protective of their kids that there are even stories of parents showing up to give professors a piece of their mind and trying to bail their kids out of bad grades and poor performances. Hofer calls these the "iConnected parents," and her advice to them is this: just let go.[2] But in today's speed-dial, text-driven world, electronic devices have become the never-ending umbilical cord between parent and child—even adult children attending college.

In an essay that appeared in the September 2015 issue of *The Atlantic*, Greg Lukianoff and Jonathan Haidt describe a related phenomenon that is happening in American colleges and universities. According to the authors, "A movement is arising, driven mostly by students, to scrub campuses clean of words, ideas and subjects that might cause discomfort and give offense."[3] Professors around the country find themselves having to teach in a more gingerly fashion for fear of eliciting a strong emotional response from the students. The student movement is about emotional well-being and presumes an extraordinary fragility in the collegiate psyche, and therefore elevates the goal of protecting students from psychological harm.

And it does appear that this generation of college students is suffering from more mental health issues than previous generations. In a 2013 survey, college mental health directors reported an across-the-board increase in the number of students with severe psychological problems.[4] It seems that the ultimate aim of this student movement, according to Lukianoff and Haidt, is to turn campuses into "safe spaces" where young adults are shielded from words and ideas that make some uncomfortable. And this movement seeks to punish anyone who interferes with that aim, even accidentally. The authors call this impulse "vindictive protectiveness." It is creating a culture in which everyone must think twice before speaking up lest they face charges of insensitivity, aggression, or worse. As Lukianoff and Haidt sum up the current situation, "Students seem to be reporting more emotional crises; many seem fragile, and this has surely changed the way university faculty and administrators interact with them. The question is whether some of those changes might be doing more harm than good."[5]

In conclusion, our devices have become such a part of our lives that we may be losing sight of who we are. We have learned to crave the endless streams of information and communication pouring in from all forms of digital media. If we want an immediate answer to something, we turn to our phone. If we need to remind our children of something or contact them, we cannot delay—we must do it now. Much of the nonstop social media and news content that we receive gets into our heads, often leading to fear, worry, and anxiety. The only way to protect our brains and the brains of our children is to become self-aware about our incessant digital communication and to make a commitment to start delaying our need for instant gratification. We must become more patient and less impulsive. This isn't impossible. We can all take steps in that direction.

CHAPTER TIPS

1. Be careful not to let the "news" take center stage in your life. Time spent surfing through the latest world crisis or political fallout is not more important than time spent with your family.

2. News organizations are competing for space in your mind. Turn off the notifications on your phone and computer and discover peace of mind instead.

3. The less time you or your children spend on social media the less exposed you will be to the world's falsehoods (fake news) and sufferings, and the less likely you will be to form the illusion that you are suffering as well.

4. Social media platforms want your attention; they want your time. They monitor everything you do and collect your data so that their algorithms can make sure you see exactly the content that you can't resist. Don't give them your time and attention; give it to your family and friends instead.

5. Let your children learn how to do things on their own. Don't do everything for them.

CHAPTER 11

Using Mindfulness and Meditation to Reconnect Our Disconnected Kids

By now I hope I have made it clear to you how technology may be adversely affecting your child and have given you a lot of good strategies to help you take back control of your child's screen time. In our final chapter together, I want to give you more help toward that goal. We're going to take a deep dive into some more unconventional but very powerful strategies that I encourage everyone to practice. But before I discuss them, I want to reiterate five core rules every parent can implement right away.

1. **Keep your child's room clean of screens.** Your child should never have any type of electronic device in their room, period. This includes televisions, computers, and handheld devices. If they tend to do

homework in the bedroom and claim they need the computer to do it, have them do it in the family room. No matter how much grief you get, remember that you are in charge. Keep those screens *out* of the bedroom.

2. **Your child's phone is your phone.** Your child's phone is yours, not theirs. Make this very clear and have a rule that the phone is to be handed to you at a certain time every night. Your child should never be allowed to sleep with the phone next to them. The temptation to communicate via text and social media throughout the night will be too strong, thereby creating sleep disturbances and other issues.

3. **No electronics during dinner.** Make a rule that dinnertime is family time. No phones or televisions can be used during this important time by anyone— including you. Make dinnertime sacred.

4. **Limit screen time for entertainment purposes (including TV) to two hours per day.** Yes, I get it, this sounds impossible, but this is what the Academy of American Pediatrics recommends for children over eight years of age. Start playing by the rules.

5. **Be a role model.** This means spending less time with your own device when you are with your children. Turn it off during dinner and whenever you are in the presence of your children. Our children need us to be present when we are around them, not distracted.

Stick to these tips and you will be well on your way to gaining control of technology in your home. Now it's time to get into some more advanced strategies to help you and your children take control of technology instead of it controlling you.

STEPPING INTO THE UNKNOWN: THE *REAL* WORLD

There is no single answer to solving the problem of modern-day screen time overdose. In a perfect world, the answer would look something like this: *just get rid of computers, smartphones, and video games.* This is obviously unrealistic. Screens and devices are here to stay, even though they have stolen a lot from our children and will continue to keep them inside and away from their friends. However, there is something that cannot be taken away from your children. You can introduce them to this powerful tool, something that will ensure they develop into fine men and women one day. It's called *thought.* You can introduce your children, and perhaps yourself, to a whole new way of thinking, an entirely new type of awareness. Let me explain.

Technology addiction, like drug addiction, strips children of their identity; they can lose sight of who they are, their sense of self. Without knowing it, their thoughts begin to control them rather than the other way around. And that's exactly how the tech industry wants it to be. Most children have never met the person who lies deep within because their time in front of screens prevents them from reflection and connection with themselves. That's going to change, because you can teach your children to get to know their inner self and become more powerful as a result. The best way to reconnect your kids to themselves is to teach them simple mental exercises, which I will get to shortly. But first we need a crash course on mindfulness.

Our mind is the result of the millions of impressions we have received from home, work, school, friends, and everything else we encounter. Nearly all of our life experiences—the things we've seen and heard, including from social media and television—are accepted by the subconscious with little or no inspection. The conscious mind receives the information and then passes it along to the subconscious, and this information is built into us mentally, emotionally, and physically. We become our thoughts. What we are today is a result of our past thinking and our past experiences. And what we become tomorrow will be the result of how we think today. It is our job to ensure that our children's minds are receiving large doses of healthy, genuine stimuli as opposed to the superficial stimuli they receive from the cyberworld.

Look at it like this: if you were planting a garden, you'd be careful to do it right. You'd buy the best soil, the best seeds, and the best sprinkler system, and you'd care for that garden so that you could grow the best crops. But when it comes to our children's mental gardens, we can be careless. What enters into their life depends on the quality of the seeds planted in their mind and how those seeds are cared for. Let's face it: if the seeds sown by social media and technology consist of gossip, fear, and a drive to keep up with the Joneses, our children's mental crop will be weak and decayed. If seeds of power, optimism, and hope are planted, cared for, and nurtured, then their mind will be resilient against any damaging thoughts received from other sources and your child's mental garden will be bountiful.

Our children have been taught their whole lives to look everywhere else but inside of themselves for answers. We never intended this, but they have become exposed to far too many negative things thanks primarily to electronic media, which has molded a mindset of lack, fear, and worry. They live in a world where they are always connected to a device and as a result disconnected from their inner selves. It is our job to create change in their environment and protect their impressionable minds. The way to do that is to teach our children how to turn inward, to connect them to their talents, desires, and dreams. Let's talk about how we can do this.

WALKING WITH A LIGHTER STEP

Regardless of the problems that clients come to me with, they all have the same thing in common: their thoughts are controlling them; they are not controlling their thoughts. I've developed an effective strategy to help my clients gain control of their thoughts and, as a result, their lives. I call it *walking with a lighter step*, and it is something you and your children can learn. Here's an illustration.

My office suite is located on the second floor of a building and faces the rear parking lot. During my initial session with clients, I ask them if they know where their car is parked. I then ask them to point it out to me from my office window. Then I ask how long they think it will take them to walk to their car after they leave my office. The answer for each person is always a little different. Some will say, "One minute." Others will say, "Forty seconds." Others might say, "Two minutes." Next, I ask this: "Let's assume that when you return for your session next week, you park in that exact same spot. How long do you think it would take you next week to walk to your car after our session has ended?" The answer is always the same as their first response. If a client said thirty seconds, they would say thirty seconds again. I then ask, "Why is this? Why wouldn't it take a little longer or be a little faster to walk to the car this time?" Their response is usually along the lines of, "I don't know; maybe because my stride is always the same," or "Because I'm a fast walker."

The purpose of this illustration is to point out that nearly everything we do throughout the day is habitual and automatic. We shower the same way, we eat our meals the same way, and we drive our cars the same way, to name just a few activities. If you eat right-handed, for example, you're not impulsively going to start eating left-handed. If you are a fast chewer you're not suddenly going to start chewing slowly. Essentially just about everything we do all day long is unconscious, meaning we don't have to "think" about what we are doing; we just do it. Something as simple as walking, whether to the car or the neighbor's house, is unconscious; we don't have to "think" about it to do it, much like riding a bike. After your brain has learned how to do something, you no longer have to try—it just happens.

I would bet that if you timed yourself daily while taking a shower, your time would always be within seconds of the previous day. The mind is a supercomputer, and once new learning is programmed into it, the brain switches to auto-pilot. This may sound like a good thing, and in some ways it is, but it is also the cause of many of our problems.

The more we go about our day "mindlessly" controlled by the subconscious, the less control we have consciously. An inner dialogue occurs during our subconscious moments, a self-talk that is unrelated to whatever mindless task we are presently engaged in, whether it's walking to the car or driving it. The mind is always wandering. It is called daydreaming, and our daydreaming thoughts are often filled with insecurities and fears. This is especially true for our children. They worry about friends, school, and what others think of them but don't realize they are doing this. The thoughts orbiting around in their subconscious universe all day long may not be positive, and the avalanche of information and images coming from social media and technology doesn't help.

It's estimated that we have approximately sixty thousand thoughts a day, most of which come from this daydreaming, subconscious mind.[1] When our thoughts are filled with worry, fear, and self-doubt, we can be sure that our life will not be as desired. Changing those subconscious daydreams requires help from the conscious, present mind. When we focus on being mentally present, we gain control of our thoughts, our body, and our emotions. Feeling our feet hitting the floor as we walk or the breath of air we are taking are exercises in self-awareness, in being present. It is from this present place that we can begin to take control of the daydreams that sabotage us.

When I ask my clients what they would need to do in order to take thirty seconds longer to walk to their car from my office, the answer is usually something like, "Walk more slowly," or "Take my time." This is true, but there is something that has to happen first before they take that first slower step. That's right: they have to catch themselves and *think* about walking more slowly. In other words, they have to become conscious. This type of conscious presence is the key to solving just about all of our problems. These present-moment awakenings, or "intentional" thoughts, remove us from the dark clouds of the subconscious, allowing us to be in command of our thoughts and therefore our feelings. Anytime we stop and think, or "stop and smell the roses," we are in a creative state because we get to paint whatever picture we want in our imagination. We can think about what we are grateful for. We can think about what we want to accomplish in life. We can think about how it feels to be motivated and confident. The more we practice present-moment, conscious thinking, the more our subconscious mind improves. Those sixty thousand drifting thoughts we have every day will begin to change, and they will begin to serve us.

Imagine you and your child going about your day and remembering as many times as you can to become mindfully present. Imagine you are at your desk, in the kitchen, or in your car, and you're catching yourself in the present moment and expanding on that present moment. Maybe you are thinking about your wonderful home and family, or maybe about being promoted or losing weight. Imagine your child sitting in the passenger seat of your car having a conversation with you because they're not distracted by a device. With practice, you and your children can start to take control of your thoughts and ultimately your outcomes.

Our thoughts become realities. When we feed our mind with thoughts of success, abundance, and confidence, eventually those thoughts make their way into the hard drive of our mind, the subconscious. And remember, it is our subconscious mind that controls about 95 percent of every aspect of us. The more we become master of our conscious, present mind, the stronger our subconscious gets. Those sixty thousand thoughts you have every day will work in your favor.

MINDFULNESS AND TECHNOLOGY

What does all of this mindfulness stuff have to do with our children's obsession with technology? Think back to your childhood for a moment. Remember those rainy days in the summer when you paced around the house trying to figure out what to do? Yes, that feeling of boredom. Well, boredom is to your brain what weightlifting is to your muscles. That's right: boredom is the mental fertilizer the mind so desperately needs. Sadly, it is something most children have never experienced.

Ask any child if they have ever sat in complete silence and paid attention to their thoughts simply because there was nothing else to do. You will find few. Kids today have no idea what boredom is because there is always an electronic device on hand to occupy them and distract them from their boredom. Unfortunately, the very thing they are distracting themselves from—their thoughts—is the thing they need the most control over in order to thrive and succeed.

Once you and your children begin to master mindfulness, there's an even faster way to start reprogramming the mind. It's called visualization. Visualization may sound clichéd, but look at it a bit differently—as a way of escaping from the distractions of technology and a way to focus your thinking. All it takes is five or ten minutes a day of your time. Start practicing visualization yourself first and then introduce it to your children. Here's a quick beginner exercise.[2]

Find a quiet place, every day, where you can sit for a few minutes in total silence completely free from all distractions, including electronic devices. Start by forming an image of something in your mind, something simple like a flower. Color that flower any color you wish. Shape the flower any way you choose. After doing this every day for a week, move on to something else that suits you, like an image of a goal that you have. For your children, maybe the image is succeeding in school or feeling determined. Make sure you breathe deeply as you do this, and stay focused on the image you have created. Remind your child to do the same. This is particularly helpful for children with anxiety, because the more they focus on images of calmness and confidence, the more quickly their mind and emotions adapt to this.

The more this is practiced, the sooner it takes root in the subconscious, which is the part of the mind that is creating how we feel all the time.

Even more important than the images your child creates while practicing this simple technique is the mental creativity they will begin to develop. This inner world is what I call the bottom of the iceberg, and the outer world is the tip. If your children practice these mental timeouts on a daily basis, they will discover that reality and personal abundance exist in their inside world, not their outer, gadget-filled world. Your children will start to feel wiser, emotionally stronger, and more in control.

THE POWER OF CONCENTRATION

Concentration is an important part of connecting to the inner self. For children this can be very difficult, because any opportunities for downtime are usually replaced with tablets and smartphones, reducing their ability to be in control of their thinking. The art of concentration is the ability to steer our mind and shape our thoughts. Doing this correctly will strengthen your child's mind and emotions.

Have your child practice this simple concentration exercise.

> Choose a specific vacation destination you've enjoyed in the past. For five minutes, close your eyes and focus all of your attention on that place—the details, the climate, the hotel, and the atmosphere. Everything.

Your child is going to find this difficult to do because their mind will wander off and think about things that have nothing to do with the vacation destination. And many of these wandering thoughts will be unpleasant. This is an example of our mind having control over us instead of us having control of it. The good news is that with regular practice your child will become a master at controlling and directing their thoughts.

Similar concentration techniques can be used to foster positive feelings. Here's one: have your child select a picture that represents a positive feeling they would like to have, such as happiness. (I like to use a picture of Rocky Balboa from the movie *Rocky* because, to me, it represents determination.) Have them stare at the picture for a few minutes, then do the following:

> Close your eyes after you've examined the picture for several minutes and try to see it vividly in your imagination. Try to see every detail. As in the first exercise, it will seem difficult to hold that picture in your thoughts for any length of time. Practice until you can see every detail for a full five minutes. Don't worry: you'll be able to do this.

Once your child has mastered this simple exercise, they will have learned the first and most important step in controlling their thoughts: concentration. This is the starting point for learning how to control feelings and attitude.

Successful athletes regularly practice similar techniques. Many experiments have been conducted with athletes to see if they can succeed at their sport by practicing their routine only in their imagination. Olympic athletes, for example, have been hooked up to sophisticated biofeedback devices that demonstrate how the same muscles that fire while competing also fire when they imagine they are competing.[3] Similar studies have been done with basketball players. One group of players was instructed to rehearse shooting free throws only in their imagination for a period of time, while the control group practiced shooting real free throws in their usual way. The group that imagined shooting free throws had the same success rate in games as the group who practiced shooting real free throws.[4] Amazing! There is no doubt our thoughts have an impact on our body and emotions. As your child practices these simple mental exercises, they will begin to see changes in how they think, feel, and act.

UNDOING ANXIETY

Ailments that we think of as "mental" often impact our physical realities. A common link to disease is anxiety. Anxiety comes directly from the subconscious, because the subconscious is like a sponge and absorbs all of the stimuli we are exposed to in the world—and there's an awful lot of it. Think about world news and all other forms of media, and how we have unintentionally given our mind free rein to wander off and absorb these messages. That's exactly why our child's subconscious can become programmed with bad stuff. It's not much different from letting your four-year-old wander off into the woods alone—it will lead to disaster.

The only way to reduce anxiety and other mental health disorders like depression is to gain mind control, and that requires focus. We only experience the ability to focus when we get into the cockpit and take over the control panels of our own mind. That's what our children must do in order to become healthy adults one day. As they learn to become mindful and apply these brief meditations, they will start to take control of their lives. Since this will likely be new to your child, mindfulness may seem a little complicated to them at first, but it isn't. It just requires practice. Your children will re-create themselves because they will be able to awaken their mind to the power within. It is imperative that you and your children practice this until you trust that the process works. I promise it will.

FAITH IN YOUR CHILD

In the 1700s, when Benjamin Franklin was studying electricity, no one believed it was real because electricity could not be seen. But although we can't see electricity, we now know it exists.[5] How else can you explain this mysterious thing that lights our homes and powers our refrigerators? Electricity is real even though we can't see it, and we have 100 percent trust in its existence. There is no disputing this. In the same way that you know about the existence of electricity, you know *you* are real. The flesh-and-blood part of you is just the host of the real *you*, also known as your mind or spirit.

You must trust that *you* are real the same way you trust that electricity is real. This is a very important part of discovering the most important relationship—the one with your *self.*

This inner self that I describe is as real as electricity. Don't believe for a minute that your powers are limited to the five senses. You are much greater than that.

Faith is generally defined as a confidence or trust in a person or entity. People use expressions such as "Have faith that everything will work out," or "I have faith in you." I think what they're really saying is, "Wake up and focus on the things you want, not on the things you don't want." The vehicle that directs our faith is the mind. If your child thinks about success, health, and abundance, they will reap the rewards of those thoughts. If they think thoughts of poverty, disease, and despair, then they will get what they wished for. Our children need to develop the faith that they are the composers of their thoughts. If they don't, they will never live up to their full potential.

· · · · ·

Our greatest gift is our ability to think. Unfortunately, many of us do not know how to do this correctly because we have relinquished this skill to screen time. But it is not too late to change. Proper thinking is the path that leads to the inner self. The inner self holds all of the answers to helping us overcome virtually anything so that we can live our lives to the fullest. The inner self is very real, and all of us have unlimited access to this world; we're just not aware of it. Those who are connected to this place are like positivity magnets, and everything they acquire in the "outside" world is a result of the work they have done inside. As you and your children practice mastering the inner self, you will all be able to balance the amount of technology in your lives and move on to greater happiness and fulfillment.

The quality of our child's life is only as good as the relationship they have with their inner self. Your child needs to learn who they truly are; they are not some superficial number based on how many "friends" or "likes" they have on social media. By applying proper mental strategies, they will discover the power of mindfulness. And if you think you could never get your child to meditate, remember the familiar phrase, "Whether you think you can or think you can't, either way you are right." So start thinking you can. After all, wouldn't you do anything for your child?

ACKNOWLEDGMENTS

I want to thank my wonderful wife, Krista, and my amazing children, Matthew and Ashlyn. I could not have done this without your love and support. You mean the world to me! I also want to thank my parents, Marge and Joe, and my siblings, Peggy, Joey, and Carrie, for being such an incredible family. I want to thank my in-laws, Tom and Phyllis, for all of their support. And finally I want to thank my great friend, Jennifer Tuma-Young, for all of the help you have provided me with over the years. And I want to thank God for being by my side and guiding me in everything I do.

NOTES

Chapter 1 Our Changing Reality

1. Gary Small, Teena D. Moody, Prabha Siddarth, and Susan Y. Bookheimer, "Your Brain on Google: Patterns of Cerebral Activation during Internet Searching," *American Journal of Geriatric Psychiatry* 17, no. 2 (2009): 116–26.

2. As quoted in Benny Evangelista, "Attention Loss Feared as High-Tech Rewires Brain," *San Francisco Chronicle*, November 15, 2009, https://www.sfgate.com/business/article/Attention-loss-feared-as-high-tech-rewires-brain-3281030.php.

3. Evangelista, "Attention Loss Feared as High-Tech Rewires Brain."

4. "29th European College of Neuropsychopharmacology (ECNP) Congress," press release, Medscape Psychiatry, September 19, 2016, https://www.medscape.com/viewcollection/33827.

5. Marion K. Underwood and Robert W. Faris, "#Being13: Inside the Secret World of Teens," CNN *Special Report*, October 2015, http://www.cnn.com/specials/us/being13.

6. Kevin P. Collins and Sean D. Cleary, "Racial and Ethnic Disparities in Parent-Reported Diagnosis of ADHD: National Survey of Children's Health (2003, 2007, and 2011)," *Journal of Clinical Psychiatry* 77, no. 1 (2016): 52–59.

7. Chaelin K. Ra et al., "Association of Digital Media Use with Subsequent Symptoms of Attention-Deficit/Hyperactivity Disorder among Adolescents," *Journal of the American Medical Association*, July 17, 2018.

8. Jean M. Twenge, Thomas E. Joiner, and Megan L. Rogers, "Increases in Depressive Symptoms, Suicide-Related Outcomes, and Suicide Rates

among U.S. Adolescents after 2010 and Links to Increased New Media Screen Time," *Clinical Psychological Science Journal*, November 14, 2017.

9. Jean M. Twenge, "The Mental Health Crisis among America's Youth Is Real—and It's Staggering," *Pennsylvania Capital-Star*, March 15, 2019, https://www.penncapital-star.com/commentary/the-mental-health-crisis-among-americas-youth-is-real-and-its-staggering-opinion/.

10. Holly Hedegaard, Sally C. Curtin, and Margaret Warner, "Suicide Mortality in the United States, 1999–2017," *National Center of Health Statistics*, Data Brief 330, November 2018.

11. All names and identifying details of clients have been changed to protect their privacy.

Chapter 2 Cyberspace Children

1. Victoria J. Rideout, Ulla G. Foehr, and Donald F. Roberts, "Generation M^2: Media in the Lives of 8- to 18-Year-Olds," A Kaiser Family Foundation Study, January 1, 2010, https://www.kff.org/other/poll-finding/report-generation-m2-media-in-the-lives/.

2. Rideout, Foehr, and Roberts, "Generation M^2."

3. Rideout, Foehr, and Roberts, "Generation M^2."

4. "Zero to Eight: Children's Media Use in America 2013," Common Sense Media, October 28, 2013, https://www.commonsensemedia.org/research/zero-to-eight-childrens-media-use-in-america-2013.

5. Veronica Rocha, "2 California Men Fall Off Edge of Ocean Bluff while Playing 'Pokemon Go'," *Los Angeles Times*, July 14, 2016, https://www.latimes.com/local/lanow/la-me-ln-pokemon-go-players-stabbed-fall-off-cliff-20160714-snap-story.html.

6. Kirstan Conley, "Many NYC Students So Tech-Oriented They Can't Even Sign Their Own Names," *New York Post*, January 27, 2016, https://nypost.com/2016/01/27/many-nyc-students-cant-even-sign-their-own-names/.

7. As quoted in Haley Goldberg, "Your Smartphone Is Making You Hallucinate," *New York Post*, January 5, 2016, https://nypost.com/2016/01/05/your-smartphone-is-making-you-hallucinate/.

8. Helena Horton, "Could You Get 'Selfie Stomach'? Internet Addict Develops Painful Disease from Hunching over Her Computer," *The Telegraph*, January 6, 2016, https://www.telegraph.co.uk/news/uknews/12084494/Selfie-addict-develops-painful-disease-from-hunching-over-her-computer.html.

9. Anthony Cuthbertson, "Smartphones Cause Drooping Jowls and 'Tech-Neck' Wrinkles in 18–39 Year-Olds," *International Business Times*, January 12, 2015, http://www.core-health.com/smartphones-cause-drooping-jowls-and-tech-neck-wrinkles-in-18-39-year-olds/.

10. As quoted in Chris Weller, "Texting Puts 50 Pounds of Pressure on Your Spine, Adding to Poor Posture's Side Effects," *Medical Daily*, November 18, 2014, https://www.medicaldaily.com/texting-puts-50 -pounds-pressure-your-spine-adding-poor-postures-side-effects-311152.

11. "Cell Phones, Wireless and Children's Health Symposium 2016: Pediatric Academic Societies," Environmental Health Trust, accessed January 21, 2020, https://ehtrust.org/science/key-scientific-lectures/cell -phones-wireless-childrens-health-symposium-2016-pediatric-societies/.

12. Melody Gutierrez, "State Kept Secret Guidelines on Safe Cell Phone Use," *San Francisco Chronicle*, March 3, 2017, https://www.sfgate .com/news/article/Judge-may-order-release-of-state-health-report-on -10973430.php.

13. Corey Egel, "CDPH Issues Guidelines on How to Reduce Exposure to Radio Frequency Energy from Cell Phones," California Department of Public Health, December 13, 2017, https://www.cdph.ca.gov/Programs /OPA/Pages/NR17-086.aspx.

14. "Channel: 5G," CTIA, accessed January 21, 2020, https://www .ctia.org/5g-channel.

15. Lori Alton, "Brain Cancer Strongly Linked to Cell Phone Radiation in Brand-New, Large-Scale Study," *NaturalHealth365*, April 19, 2018, https://www.naturalhealth365.com/brain-cancer-emf-2532.html.

16. Alton, "Brain Cancer Strongly Linked to Cell Phone Radiation."

17. Alton, "Brain Cancer Strongly Linked to Cell Phone Radiation."

18. Jeromy Johnson, "Smart Cities, 5G and EMF Pollution: How This 'New' Technology Will INCREASE Our Exposure to Microwave Radiation," *NaturalHealth365*, June 18, 2017, https://www.naturalhealth365 .com/emf-wireless-technology-2278.html.

19. Johnson, "Smart Cities, 5G and EMF Pollution."

20. Johnson, "Smart Cities, 5G and EMF Pollution."

21. Johnson, "Smart Cities, 5G and EMF Pollution."

22. Jennifer McGraw, "Parents Blame Elementary School's Cell Tower after 4th Student Diagnosed with Cancer," March 12, 2019, https://sacra mento.cbslocal.com/2019/03/12/school-cell-tower-causing-cancer.

23. McGraw, "Parents Blame Elementary School's Cell Tower."

24. Josh del Sol Beaulieu, "Brussels Says No to 5G," *Collective Evolution*, April 2, 2019.

25. Beaulieu, "Brussels Says No to 5G."

26. Beaulieu, "Brussels Says No to 5G."

27. Elizabeth Aguilera, "Too Much 'Brexting' Undermines Bonding during Breastfeeding," KPCC, September 24, 2015, https://www.scpr .org/news/2015/09/24/54595/brexting-impacts-baby-bonding-during -breastfeeding.

Chapter 3 Social Media and the Development of Self-Esteem

1. "From 'I Hate You' to 'Thank You'—Abby Jones—TEDxCherry CreekWomen," YouTube Video, 9:37, uploaded by TEDx Talks, December 12, 2018, https://www.youtube.com/watch?v=c_0dJJhIrSo.

2. Underwood and Faris, "#Being13: Inside the Secret World of Teens."

3. Susan Kelley, "'Likes' Less Likely to Affect Self-Esteem of People with Purpose," *Cornell Chronicle*, September 21, 2016, https://news.cornell.edu/stories/2016/09/likes-less-likely-affect-self-esteem-people-purpose.

4. Jean M. Twenge, Zlatan Krizan, and Garrett Hisler, "Decreases in Self-Reported Sleep Duration among U.S. Adolescents 2009–2015 and Association with New Media Screen Time," *Sleep Medicine* 39 (November 2017): 47–53.

5. Sabrina Tavernise, "Young Adolescents as Likely to Die from Suicide as from Traffic Accidents," *New York Times*, November 3, 2016, https://www.nytimes.com/2016/11/04/health/suicide-adolescents-traffic-deaths.html.

6. As quoted in Tavernise, "Young Adolescents as Likely to Die from Suicide."

Chapter 4 The Multitasking Brains of Kids

1. Melina R. Uncapher and Anthony D. Wagner, "Minds and Brains of Media Multitaskers: Current Findings and Future Directions," *Proceedings of the National Academy of Sciences of the United States of America* 115, no. 40 (October 2, 2018): 9889–96.

2. Eyal Ophir, Clifford Nass, and Anthony D. Wagner, "Cognitive Control in Media Multitaskers," *Proceedings of the National Academy of Sciences of the United States of America* 106, no. 37 (September 15, 2009): 15583–87.

3. Sanjay Gupta, "Your Brain on Multitasking," *CNN Health*, August 1, 2016, http://www.cnn.com/2015/04/09/health/your-brain-multitasking.

4. Small, Moody, Siddarth, and Bookheimer, "Your Brain on Google."

5. Travis Bradberry, "Multitasking Damages Your Brain and Your Career, New Studies Suggest," *Talentsmart Newsletter*, accessed December 9, 2019, http://www.talentsmart.com/articles/Multitasking-Damages-Your-Brain-and-Your-Career,-New-Studies-Suggest-2102500909-p-1.html.

6. Jeff Guo, "Why Smart Kids Shouldn't Use Laptops in Class," *Washington Post*, May 18, 2016.

7. Guo, "Why Smart Kids Shouldn't Use Laptops in Class."

8. Guo, "Why Smart Kids Shouldn't Use Laptops in Class."

9. James Doubek, "Attention, Students: Put Your Laptops Away," *NPR Weekend Edition*, April 17, 2016, https://www.npr.org/2016/04/17/474525392/attention-students-put-your-laptops-away.

10. Anderson Cooper, "Groundbreaking Study Examines Effects of Screen Time on Kids," *60 Minutes*, December 9, 2018, https://www.cbs news.com/news/groundbreaking-study-examines-effects-of-screen-time -on-kids-60-minutes/.

11. Cooper, "Groundbreaking Study Examines Effects of Screen Time on Kids."

12. Cooper, "Groundbreaking Study Examines Effects of Screen Time on Kids."

13. Richard B. Lopez, Todd F. Heatherton, and Dylan D. Wagner, "Media Multitasking: Using Multiple Digital Devices at Same Time Linked to Obesity," *Brain Imaging and Behavior*, March 1, 2019, https://link .springer.com/article/10.1007/s11682-019-00056-0#citeas.

14. Lopez, Heatherton, and Wagner, "Media Multitasking."

Chapter 5 Gamer Kids

1. Tom Phillips, "Taiwan Orders Parents to Limit Children's Time with Electronic Games," *The Telegraph*, January 28, 2015, https://www .telegraph.co.uk/news/worldnews/asia/taiwan/11373521/Taiwan-orders -parents-to-limit-childrens-time-with-electronic-games.html.

2. Tom Phillips, "Chinese Teen Chops Hand Off to 'Cure' Internet Addiction," *The Telegraph*, February 3, 2015, https://www.telegraph .co.uk/news/worldnews/asia/china/11386325/Chinese-teen-chops-hand -off-to-cure-internet-addiction.html.

3. "Stories of Video Game Addiction—Straight from the Horse's Mouth," Video Game Addiction, accessed December 10, 2019, http://www.video -game-addiction.org/stories-of-addiction.html.

4. James Batchelor, "Global Games Market Value Rising to 134.9bn in 2018," gamesindustry.biz, December 18, 2018, https://www.games industry.biz/articles/2018-12-18-global-games-market-value-rose-to-usd 134-9bn-in-2018.

5. Jeff Glor, "'Gaming Disorder' Recognized as a Mental Health Condition by World Health Organization," CBS News, June 18, 2018, https:// www.cbsnews.com/news/compulsive-video-game-playing-world-health -organization/.

6. Glor, "'Gaming Disorder' Recognized as a Mental Health Condition."

7. John Raphael, "Study: How Videogame Addiction Affects Sleep Habits, Obesity, Cardio-Metabolic Health," *Nature World News*, May 11, 2016, https://www.natureworldnews.com/articles/21883/20160511 /study-videogame-addiction-affects-sleep-habits-obesity-cardio-meta bolic-health.htm.

Chapter 6 Parenting from a Distance

1. Norman Herr, "Television & Health," Internet Resources to Accompany *The Sourcebook for Teaching Science*, accessed November 16, 2016, http://www.csun.edu/science/health/docs/tv&health.html.

2. "American Academy of Pediatrics Announces New Recommendations for Children's Media Use," American Academy of Pediatrics, October 21, 2016, https://www.aap.org/en-us/about-the-aap/aap-press-room/Pages/American-Academy-of-Pediatrics-Announces-New-Recommendations-for-Childrens-Media-Use.aspx.

3. Linda S. Pagani, Marie Josee Harbec, and Tracie A. Barnett, "Prospective Associations between Television in the Preschool Bedroom and Later Bio-Psycho-Social Risks," *Pediatric Research* 85, no. 7 (December 26, 2018): 967–73.

4. Sarah Myruski et al., "Digital Disruption? Maternal Mobile Device Use Is Related to Infant Social-Emotional Functioning," *Developmental Science* 21, no. 4 (July 2018): e12610.

5. "Technology Addiction: Concern, Controversy, and Finding Balance," Common Sense Media, May 2016, https://www.commonsensemedia.org/research/technology-addiction-concern-controversy-and-finding-balance.

6. "Technology Addiction."

7. "1 in 3 Can't Get through Meal without Looking at Phone, Survey Finds," Study Finds, February 15, 2018, https://www.studyfinds.org/phone-eating-meal-distracted/.

8. Josh Hafner, "Child Drownings Linked to Phone-Distracted Parents Who Fail to Look Up," *USA Today*, August 15, 2018, https://www.usatoday.com/story/news/nation-now/2018/08/15/child-drownings-linked-phone-distraction-among-parents-pools/998836002/.

9. Hafner, "Child Drownings Linked to Phone-Distracted Parents."

10. Associated Press, "Would You Do a Phone-Free Holiday? Growing Number of Hotels Are Offering Free Perks to Guests—but They Must Hand Over Their Devices," *Daily Mail*, December 21, 2018, https://www.dailymail.co.uk/travel/travel_news/article-6518973/Digital-detox-Resorts-offer-perks-handing-phones.html.

11. Janet Morrissey, "Your Phone's on Lockdown. Enjoy the Show," *New York Times*, October 16, 2016, https://www.nytimes.com/2016/10/16/technology/your-phones-on-lockdown-enjoy-the-show.html.

Chapter 7 How Handheld Devices Impact Emotional Development

1. "Emotional Intelligence: Mixed Model," Universal Class, accessed December 10, 2019, https://www.universalclass.com/articles/psychology/emotional-intelligence-mixed-model.htm.

2. Peter Gray, "Declining Student Resilience: A Serious Problem for Colleges," *Psychology Today*, September 22, 2015, https://www.psychology today.com/us/blog/freedom-learn/201509/declining-student-resilience -serious-problem-colleges.

3. Gray, "Declining Student Resilience."

4. "Are You Multitasking Your Life Away? Cliff Nass at TEDx Stanford," YouTube video, 2:23, uploaded by TEDx Talks, June 20, 2013, https://www.youtube.com/watch?v=PriSFBu5CLs.

5. Collin Binkley, "Colleges' Message to Ease Student Stress: Failure Is Normal," April 4, 2019, *AP News*, https://www.apnews.com/c6bde0 dd123a4b81a2388d3c28830a24.

6. Binkley, "Colleges' Message to Ease Student Stress."

7. Ben Locke et al., "Center for Collegiate Mental Health: 2015 Annual Report," Penn State University, accessed January 21, 2020, https://sites .psu.edu/ccmh/files/2017/10/2015_CCMH_Report_1-18-2015-yq3vik.pdf.

8. "American College Health Association National College Health Assessment: Fall 2017 Reference Group Executive Summary," ACHA, accessed January 21, 2020, https://www.acha.org/documents/ncha/NCHA -II_FALL_2017_REFERENCE_GROUP_EXECUTIVE_SUMMARY.pdf.

9. Roy Pea et al., "Media Use, Face-to-Face Communication, Media Multitasking, and Social Well-Being among 8–12-Year-Old Girls," *Developmental Psychology* 48, no. 2 (2012): 327–36.

10. Pea et al., "Media Use."

11. Piush Mandhane, "Screen-Time Is Associated with Inattention Problems in Preschoolers: Results from the CHILD Birth Cohort Study," *Plos One* (April 17, 2019): e0213995.

12. University of Alberta Faculty of Medicine & Dentistry, "Screen Time Associated with Behavioral Problems in Preschoolers," *Medical Xpress*, April 17, 2019, https://medicalxpress.com/news/2019-04-screen -behavioral-problems-preschoolers.html.

13. American Academy of Pediatrics, "Handheld Screen Time Linked with Speech Delays in Young Children," *EurekAlert!*, May 4, 2017, https:// www.eurekalert.org/pub_releases/2017-05/aaop-hst042617.php.

14. American Academy of Pediatrics, "Handheld Screen Time Linked."

Chapter 8 The Digital Classroom

1. OECD, "Students, Computers and Learning: Making the Connection," *OECDiLibrary*, September 15, 2015, https://read.oecd-ilibrary.org /education/students-computers-and-learning_9789264239555-en.

2. Eliane Glaser, "Children Are Tech Addicts—and Schools Are the Pushers," *The Guardian*, January 26, 2018, https://www.theguardian .com/commentisfree/2018/jan/26/children-tech-addicts-schools.

3. Glaser, "Children Are Tech Addicts."

4. Jason Rogers, Alex Usher, and Edyta Kaxnowska, "The State of E-Learning in Canadian Universities, 2011: If Students Are Digital Natives, Why Don't They Like E-Learning?" Higher Education Strategy Associates, September 2011, https://higheredstrategy.com/wp-content/uploads/2011/09/InsightBrief42.pdf.

5. Sean Cavanagh, "Amazon, Apple, Google, and Microsoft Battle for K-12 Market, and Loyalties of Educators," *Edweek Market Brief*, May 8, 2017, https://marketbrief.edweek.org/special-report/amazon-apple-google-and-microsoft-battle-for-k-12-market-and-loyalties-of-educators/.

6. Cavanagh, "Amazon, Apple, Google, and Microsoft."

7. Natasha Singer and Danielle Ivory, "How Silicon Valley Plans to Conquer the Classroom," *New York Times*, November 3, 2017, https://www.nytimes.com/2017/11/03/technology/silicon-valley-baltimore-schools.html.

8. Singer and Ivory, "How Silicon Valley Plans."

9. Singer and Ivory, "How Silicon Valley Plans."

10. Singer and Ivory, "How Silicon Valley Plans."

Chapter 9 Raising Our Children to Be Leaders Instead of Followers

1. As quoted in Zoe W. Linza, "NABE President's Message—March 2017," NABE, accessed January 21, 2020, https://www.nabenet.org/page/NABENewsMar2017Prez.

Chapter 10 Fragile Kids

1. "Booing Banned in Some New England Soccer Matches," LinkedIn SlideShare, accessed January 21, 2020, https://www.slideshare.net/Eyalyechezkell/booing-banned-in-some-new-england-soccer-matches.

2. Barbara K. Hofer and Abigail Sullivan Moore, *The iConnected Parent: Staying Close to Your Kids in College (and Beyond) While Letting Them Grow Up* (New York: Atria Books, 2010).

3. Greg Lukianoff and Jonathan Haidt, "The Coddling of the American Mind," *The Atlantic*, September 2015, https://www.theatlantic.com/magazine/archive/2015/09/the-coddling-of-the-american-mind/399356/.

4. Gray, "Declining Student Resilience."

5. Lukianoff and Haidt, "The Coddling of the American Mind."

Chapter 11 Using Mindfulness and Meditation to Reconnect Our Disconnected Kids

1. Remez Sasson "How Many Thoughts Does Your Mind Think in One Hour?" Success Consciousness, accessed January 21, 2020, https://

www.successconsciousness.com/blog/inner-peace/how-many-thoughts
-does-your-mind-think-in-one-hour/.

2. You can also go to my website, www.tomkersting.com, to receive
an audio version of the exercise.

3. Ken Johnston, "The Olympics, Then . . . Now . . . and the Edge,"
Creating Positive Change (blog), February 28, 2010, http://freshaire
creatingpositivechange.blogspot.com/2010/02/olympics-thennowand
-edge.html.

4. Joe Haefner, "Mental Rehearsal & Visualization: The Secret to Im-
proving Your Game without Touching a Basketball!" Breakthrough Basketball, accessed November 16, 2016, https://www.breakthroughbasket
ball.com/mental/visualization.html.

5. This illustration is taken from Rhonda Byrne, *The Secret* (New
York: Atria Books, 2006).

Tom Kersting is a nationally renowned psychotherapist, and retired high school counselor. He appears regularly on popular talk shows and news shows and has also hosted television series and shows for A&E Network, National Geographic Channel, Food Network, and Oprah's Wellness Network. He lectures throughout the country and hosts the *Reconnected Parent* podcast. He maintains a busy counseling practice in New Jersey.

CONNECT WITH TOM

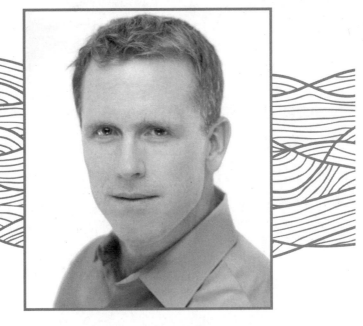

TOMKERSTING.COM

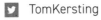 TomKersting   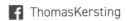 ThomasKersting

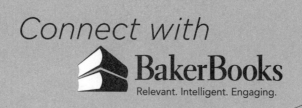
 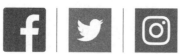